Disabled Childhoods

T0331478

A crucial contemporary dynamic around children and young people in the Global North is the multiple ways that have emerged to monitor their development, behaviour and character. In particular, disabled children or children with unusual developmental patterns can find themselves surrounded by multiple practices through which they are examined.

This rich book draws on a wide range of qualitative research to look at how disabled children have been cared for, treated and categorised. Narrative and longitudinal interviews with children and their families, along with stories and images they have produced, and notes from observations of different spaces in their lives – medical consultation rooms, cafes and leisure centres, homes, classrooms and playgrounds amongst others – all make a contribution.

Bringing this wealth of empirical data together with conceptual ideas from disability studies, sociology of the body, childhood studies, symbolic interactionism and feminist critical theory, the authors explore the multiple ways in which monitoring occurs within childhood disability and the social effects of this monitoring. Their discussion includes examining the dynamics of differentiation via medicine, social interaction and embodiment, and the multiple actors – including children and young people themselves – involved. The book also investigates the practices that differentiate children into different categories and what this means for notions of normality, integration, belonging and citizenship.

Scrutinising the multiple forms of monitoring around disabled children, and the consequences they generate for how we think about childhood and what is 'normal', this volume sits at the intersection of disability studies and childhood studies.

Janice McLaughlin is a Professor at the University of Newcastle, UK, and the Subject Head of Sociology. She researches childhood disability with a particular focus on family life, and on the social implications of medical intervention and diagnosis. She works across disability studies, social and medical anthropology, and childhood/youth studies in order to understand the multiple factors shaping childhood and disability, and the role of children themselves in shaping their lives. There is a strong focus on the significance of social interaction, narrative and embodiment in the development and maintenance of identity, but this is mediated by a need to consider questions of inequality, marginalisation and injustice.

Edmund Coleman-Fountain is a Research Fellow in the Social Policy Research Unit at the University of York. He received his PhD in sociology from Newcastle University in 2011 after which he worked in the Policy, Ethics and Life Sciences Research Centre. His research has focused on questions of difference, citizenship and equality in the identity narratives of lesbian and gay youths and disabled youths. His publications include *Understanding Narrative Identity through Lesbian and Gay Youth* (Palgrave Macmillan, 2014).

Emma Clavering is currently a Teaching Fellow in Sociology at the School of Geography, Politics and Sociology at Newcastle University. Her key research interests explore narratives of social and cultural identity in everyday worlds of family, kinship and self, with particular focus on consumer culture, particularly in relation to embodiment and notions of health and difference. She is a co-author, along with Janice McLaughlin, of *Families Raising Disabled Children: Enabling Care and Social Justice* (Palgrave 2008).

Routledge Advances in Disability Studies

Disabled Childhoods

Monitoring differences and emerging identities

**Janice McLaughlin,
Edmund Coleman-Fountain
and Emma Clavering**

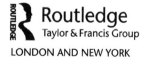

Routledge
Taylor & Francis Group

LONDON AND NEW YORK

First published 2016
by Routledge
2 Park Square, Milton Park, Abingdon, Oxon OX14 4RN

and by Routledge
711 Third Avenue, New York, NY 10017

First issued in paperback 2017

Routledge is an imprint of the Taylor & Francis Group, an informa business

British Library Cataloguing-in-Publication Data
A catalogue record for this book is available from the British Library

Library of Congress Cataloging-in-Publication Data
McLaughlin, Janice, 1968– , author.
Disabled childhoods : monitoring differences and emerging identities /
Janice McLaughlin, Edmund Coleman-Fountain, and Emma Clavering.
    p. ; cm. – (Routledge advances in disability studies)
    Includes bibliographical references and index.
    ISBN 978-0-415-74974-9 (hbk) – ISBN 978-1-315-79589-8 (ebk)
    I. Coleman-Fountain, Edmund, author. II. Clavering, Emma, author.
    III. Title. IV. Series: Routledge advances in disability studies.
    [DNLM: 1. Developmental Disabilities–Europe. 2. Developmental
    Disabilities–North America. 3. Disabled Children–Europe. 4. Disabled
    Children–North America. 5. Adolescent–Europe. 6. Adolescent–North
    America. 7. Child–Europe. 8. Child–North America. 9. Social Norms–
    Europe. 10. Social Norms–North America. WS 350.6]
    RJ506.D47
    362.2–dc23   2015034344

ISBN 13: 978-1-138-49450-3 (pbk)
ISBN 13: 978-0-415-74974-9 (hbk)

Typeset in Times New Roman
by Wearset Ltd, Boldon, Tyne and Wear

To a good colleague and friend: Jackie Leach Scully

Contents

PART IV
Implications 159

Figures

Introduction

The current lives of, and possibilities for, disabled children and young people in much of the Global North bear little resemblance to the lives of those born in earlier generations. They are more likely to live at home with their families rather than be placed in institutions, to be in mainstream schools, to have access to many aspects of the public sphere, to have options about living independently in adulthood, to go into higher education and move on to careers (Anaby et al., 2013; Beckett, 2009; Lindsay and McPherson, 2012; Shields et al., 2012). Changes in medical diagnosis and treatment, alongside other socio-economic changes, also mean that those with some of the most serious life-threatening and -shortening disabling conditions are also living longer, and living longer while participants in society (Knapp et al., 2008; Mitchell, 2014). However, there are several reasons to still query the social position of disabled children and young people and to explore contemporary dynamics of marginalisation and exclusion. Disabled children and young people and their families continue to report a range of difficulties created by community dislike and hostility towards them, by battles with welfare agencies to have their needs recognised and supported, and by significant financial difficulties created by the overlapping effects of additional care costs, drops in family income, and decline in welfare provision (Atkinson et al., 2015; Goodley and Runswick-Cole, 2011). While our work is centred in the UK, research across different global capitalist economies has identified similar patterns in the context of changes in welfare provision, social attitudes and capitalist strategies (Parish, 2013; Spencer and Strazdins, 2015). Draw this further out to disabled children and young people in the varied locations of the Global South, and again a complex picture emerges of greater international and state recognition of their rights to a good quality of life, alongside massive problems created by deep economic insecurity, state vulnerabilities, environmental destruction and armed conflict (Bühler-Niederberger and Van Krieken, 2005; Plan International, 2013; UNICEF, 2013).

When a child is identified as having differences in their functioning and development they are drawn into a cycle of institutional intervention and support. This support and aid is an important reason why children born with or who acquire a range of impairments are now living longer and reporting a better quality of life. However, the intervention and support received, combined with the differences in their minds-bodies that bring them to the attention of such help, also mark them out as distinct from other children. Children and young people vary in all sorts of ways – they differ in how they look, move and act, in how they develop, and in their social background. What we are interested in is the ways in which children and young people with differences in their minds-bodies that society marks out as disability become situated as other, through the ways in which those differences are identified, defined and responded to. In doing so, we are not saying it is just the operation of categorisation that produces disability; instead it is how the differences that become categorised as disability interact with those processes of categorisation that produce a life that in some aspects is disabled. That is, we want to resist a move to see what we are examining as only a discursive process. We aim to bring social practice and discursive framing together through an interest in what people do, as well as what they narrate as being significant. There are several benefits of maintaining an interest in social practice and interaction, alongside discursive social constructions that help frame our identity and social position. First, children and young people maintain a presence as active in responding to both the worlds they are part of and the minds-bodies they are in. We stay attuned to the moments of agency, resistance, and altered imaginaries that they are participating in creating. Second, it avoids a consideration only of institutional structures or everyday relationships by exploring how people interact within key institutions of contemporary life. Third, it aids us to explore how ways of being and social organisation are maintained in ways that marginalise and generate othering, while also enabling us to identify resistant possibilities. Finally, it connects a focus on practice and discourse to considerations of citizenship and rights by asking what are the multiple factors in inhibiting access to citizenship. First, in terms of being able to participate in the practices of citizenship, and second, in being recognised as a person who is a valued citizen.

Therefore, we are interested in both formal processes of differentiation that occur through key institutions such as medicine and education, alongside the everyday practices of social life that help demarcate differences in particular ways. Our argument is that as disabled children and young people (and we will come back to this category in a moment) have been integrated into society more fully, and found a presence in their social worlds, that the ways in which their differences continue to be notable matter to their position, identities and future possibilities. They are notable through both modes of classifying those differences and also through how they are part of social interaction with others. This is what we mean by 'monitoring' – the multiple ways in which particular differences in child and adolescent bodies are observed, categorised, and classified, and the ways in which those monitoring practices matter politically. One product of monitoring is the maintenance of boundaries between normal and abnormal minds-bodies and children and young people. The politics of complete seclusion of disabled children and young people to the hidden margins of society has been replaced by the, perhaps more subtle, ways in which judgements and comparisons are made between them and others said to be normal. Our concern, to match the times, is with the contemporary policing and disciplinary dynamics faced by disabled children and young people, and how they themselves engage with such dynamics. We believe that this is an important way to explore contemporary childhood, not just as a way to understand the lives of disabled children and young people, but because of what it says more broadly about how children are policed in contemporary society. In particular, what it says about the complex processes through which children and young people are ascribed identities, which draw from values of normality and ordinariness, but also how they challenge and resist such ascriptions in their own enactments and explorations of identity in the context of difference.

Our book draws from a number of research projects we have undertaken, alongside a range of conceptual tools we use to think about the contemporary modes of monitoring, surveillance and resistance that disabled children and young people participate in. Before outlining how we will do that across the structure of the book, there are a few key terms we first need to clarify.

What is disability and who are disabled children and young people?

There are different frameworks for defining children and young people as disabled; each way of producing the categorisation brings with it different approaches to understanding what is signified by disability and, subsequently, how those then placed within the category should be responded to. We summarise these here in order to clarify how we are using the phrase, but the frameworks introduced will be fully explored in the book itself. The first route to define disability is through the formal classifications produced by medicine. Medicine categorises a range of embodied differences as being some kind of distinctive human condition and child development. These categories (while not being sufficient in themselves) are then drawn upon by the state to decide whether someone has the right to welfare support and legal protection. Both the state and medicine focus on what is distinctive about the individual and then classify types of distinctive individual into different categories of limitation and deficit. Their response is to then treat those limitations and seek to make up the deficit within the individual.

A second way to think about disability has emerged from political dissatisfaction with these formal categories and measures. The disability movement and disability studies in the UK developed the social model in order to make a distinction between impairment – the things wrong with the body (and in some definitions the mind) – and disability – the things wrong with society that make it difficult for those with impairments to participate to the same level as others (UPIAS, 1976). People's bodies can differ in lots of ways, including capacity, but that difference becomes a disability when the organisation of society makes it more difficult to participate. Therefore the deficit or limitation is no longer embodied in the individual – it is in the social structure and it is that which requires fixing. While the social model began with a focus on material problems such as physical access to the public sphere, it has increasingly also been concerned with social attitudes as important in marginalising disabled people. The social model has opened up understandings of disability and created greater appreciation of how the category is a social and political one, which places the gaze upon society, rather than the individual (Barton, 1996, 2001). It has been adapted and revised by a number of writers, in part to engage more with questions relating to non-physical impairments such as learning styles and mental well-being, but also to engage in more experiential and emotional aspects of living in a society that fails to adapt to the ways in which people's minds-bodies may differ from the norm (Shakespeare, 2006; Shakespeare and Watson, 2001; Thomas, 2004a, 2004b). However, more recently, a range of writers have advocated for further revision in how we think about disability, which expands once more our understanding of the category. Such writers place equal social scrutiny on the category of impairment itself (Goodley, 2001). In particular, critical disability studies returns to the categories of medicine and the state to argue that the problem is not just that they do not focus on the real problem – the unwelcoming nature of society – but that they are also productive of disability itself through their categorisation of impairment. That by turning different embodied attributes into different medical labels they produce different categories of person.

    Our consideration of disabled childhoods shares much with the conceptual expansion that has enabled an interrogation of institutionalised approaches to disability's definition and use. We are interested in the lack of fit between society and children and young people with minds-bodies that differ from the norm. Therefore, when we use the phrase disabled children and young people we refer to children and young people whose minds-bodies interact with the world in a different way; a difference that places them in recognised categories, established in medicine, validated by state institutions, and maintained by how others in society, known and unknown, engage with them. Disability is therefore emergent in a range of social and institutional experiences that children with a range of embodied differences will have. 'Disabled childhoods' we use to reflect the influence of broader norms of childhood and adolescence in shaping the disabling practices and discourses disabled children and young people encounter. To emphasise the social quality of the term disabled children and young people we could have used scare quotes or a different term. For example, we did explore using Holt's (2004) formulation of children with mind-body differences, due to how it brings together embodied experience, with broader socio-economic conditions. The phrasing is also valuable because it uses the hyphenated 'mind-body' to blur the Cartesian mind and body split (at times we do use this to acknowledge the mix of differences a child can enact that are the subject of societal and institutional scrutiny). However, we have opted to remain, for the most part, with the category of disabled children and young people. This is for two main reasons; first, we maintain the use of the phrase to position our arguments as within the continuum of work established in the social model and critical disability studies. Crucially, that the disability is not in the person (therefore not using 'person with'), but in the gap between society and the person. While we approach this gap differently from the various accounts of the social model and critical disability studies, there is a political value in emphasising the debt and allegiance owed to that rich body of work and activism. Second, a somewhat more pragmatic one we acknowledge, is the greater readability of the phrase over more nuanced configurations of terms. Likewise, our exploration of disabled childhoods includes the distinctive landscape of adolescence, but we refer to disabled childhoods rather than disabled childhoods and adolescence for brevity. Reference to childhood studies also is used to include youth studies as a sub-group of that broader work.

Although we use the disabled children and young people phrase, we should also acknowledge the limitations embedded in the term. First, emphasising the social production of disability should not be at the cost of failing to acknowledge that aspects of living in a mind-body which differs in capacity can produce limitations (Scully, 2008). For example, significant pain and/or a shortened life. The differences that a specific mind-body makes to someone's life is not just what comes from the outside world. Second, we are not suggesting the experiences of those whose social position places them in the category of 'disabled' will be uniform. Again our focus is on understanding how living in a mind-body that places you within certain categories of difference, here focused on disability, will generate a range of experiences to make sense of and navigate through. Finally, for those within the disability category there are a range of other embodied variations that also matter to them and to their social positioning. Within the category of child and young person there are significant variations relating to age (not necessarily in an incremental developmental sense) and other key aspects of their social background and location which, through a series of interactions, will shape their lives. Across the book the intent is that we do not lose sight of these complexities and contingencies in understanding the socially sophisticated lives of those within the category of disabled children and young people. At certain points we speak of children, rather than children and young people – this is when the dynamics being explored are more associated with the stages of childhood associated with pre-adolescence.

One final thing it is important we acknowledge here is that our research has occurred in the Global North, and this location does lead to a privileging of that location within our analysis. However, we do at times (perhaps not enough), draw other locations into the account to both acknowledge the situated nature of our positioning (Bühler-Niederberger and Van Krieken, 2005; Greenfield, 2009; Kagitcibasi, 1996) and to draw parallels between different locations and experiences.

Outline of the book

The book focus and structure is influenced by two things. First, the book is an accumulation of a decade of empirical research on disabled childhoods. This means that the data we have gathered, and our interpretation of it, is a strong influence on the themes of the book. Second, we have divided the book into four parts:

- Part I: Theoretical and methodological practices
- Part II: Monitoring institutions
- Part III: Relational identity and practice
- Part IV: Implications

The first part lays out the theoretical tools we draw from and the production of the data that is also central to our discussions. Parts II and III capture an analytical distinction we are making. Our interest, as will become clearer in Chapter 1, is in how monitoring is something that works across both what formal institutions do, and also what happens within the everyday worlds of interaction and identity. These are not separate processes, institutions are informed by interaction, and interaction is informed by institutions. So while Part II focuses on key institutions of monitoring and Part III on key relational dynamics, the account will also highlight the interaction between these two fields of activity. The final part moves away from an account of the data to think through, conceptually and politically, what the different patterns of monitoring mean for how we think through the citizenship of disabled children and young people – now and into the future.

In a little more detail the chapters do the following.

Chapter 1: Theorising disabled childhoods

The book creates a bridge between childhood studies, youth studies and disability studies; this chapter explains how we make that bridge and why. Through the discussion, it makes the case for why childhood studies should pay more attention to disability, and why disability studies should pay more attention to how childhood and adolescence (and the transitions between) emerge within social relations and institutions. We also outline how and why we draw from a range of other conceptual sources in the book: in particular, embodiment studies, symbolic interactionism and social studies of technology.

Chapter 2: Methodological approaches

Here we explore the development of the different methodological approaches we have used to explore childhood via work with parents, carers (formal and informal), broader family members, and children and young people themselves. Within the umbrella of ethnography we will discuss techniques such as narrative interviews, observation, visual methods and creative practice. We also discuss key current debates about how distinctive methods should be for working with children and young people, and the contemporary important agenda around participatory methods.

Chapter 3: Institutional norms and transitions

A key concept in the book is the manufacture of notions of normality as an ideal against which people are judged and categorised depending on their difference from it. This chapter looks at key institutions where such norms are established. In particular, education and then the subsequent transition to the institutions of adulthood: higher education, work and family. We explore in these different settings the policing qualities of norms of being, and the work that disabled children and young people embark on to approximate them.

Chapter 4: Engagements with medical diagnosis and intervention

Medicine is an important vehicle for the production of templates of child development, definitions of disability and its treatment, and boundaries between normality and abnormality. This chapter engages with how medicine comes to play this role within childhood disability, but in a way that does not assume that medicine's authority is absolute. Instead we consider how people's existing sources of understanding their identity and others' interact with the meanings produced by medicine to shape its influence. Particular focus is given to genetics in order to consider how much significance we can, or should, give to it as a contemporary meta-narrative capable of redefining human variation into forms of medical disorder.

Chapter 5: Embodied practices and valued identities

Embodiment studies has not done much work within the contexts of disability, particularly within childhood, but it is important to consider disabled children as embodied actors, making use of their bodies in their complex identity negotiations. This chapter looks at such practices and their implications for how we think about patterns of marginalisation and exclusion, but also of creative relational agency. We pay particular attention to the multiple influences on how disabled children and young people engage with their bodies, enabling us to again show how medicine is not the only factor influencing meaning and practice, and also how other social factors such as gender intersect in body work related to monitoring disability.

Chapter 6: Making family

Families are not the only relationships that children and young people are part of, but nevertheless the varied family forms that children and young people are within are important contexts to their lives. This chapter looks at how disabled children and young people are, and are not, within their family, and how notions such as resemblance, inheritance, care and good parenting play a part in the creation of family ties – ties the child/young person is part of creating. It will also look at the multiple forms of scrutiny families with 'different' children fall under and how families manage such scrutiny.

Chapter 7: Embodied and relational citizenship

We conclude the book by examining the implications of our discussions of monitoring through the lens of citizenship. This is done because of the way in which citizenship brings together our interest in institutional practices of monitoring, with everyday relational dynamics of identity recognition and mis-recognition. We look at current requirements of citizenship in both adulthood – being normal – and in childhood – having capacity – in order to problematize the conditions that the contemporary neo-liberal state and society place on being recognised as a citizen and having the rights to participate in society.

References

Anaby, D., Hand, C., Bradley, L., DiRezze, B., Forhan, M., DiGiacomo, A. and Law, M. (2013) The effect of the environment on participation of children and youth with disabilities: a scoping review. *Disability and Rehabilitation*, 35(19): 1589–1598.

Atkinson, M., Rees, D. and Davis, L. (2015) Disability and economic disadvantage: facing the facts. *Archives of Disease in Childhood*, 100(4): 305–307.

Barton, L. (ed.) (1996) *Disability and Society: Emerging Issues and Insights*. London: Longman.

Barton, L. (ed.) (2001) *Disability Politics and the Struggle for Change*. London: David Fulton.

Beckett, A.E. (2009) 'Challenging disabling attitudes, building an inclusive society': considering the role of education in encouraging non-disabled children to develop positive attitudes towards disabled people. *British Journal of Sociology of Education*, 30(3): 317–329.

Bühler-Niederberger, D. and Van Krieken, R. (2005) Persisting inequalities: childhood between global influences and local traditions. *Childhood*, 15(2): 147–155.

Goodley, D. (2001) 'Learning difficulties', the social model of disability and impairment: challenging epistemologies. *Disability & Society*, 16(2): 207–231.

Goodley, D. and Runswick-Cole, K. (2011) The violence of disablism. *Sociology of Health and Illness*, 33(4): 602–617.

Greenfield, P.M. (2009) Independence and interdependence as developmental scripts. In P.M. Greenfield and R.R. Cocking (eds.), *Cultural Roots of Minority Child Development*. pp. 1–39. Hillside, NJ: Erlbaum.

Holt, L. (2004) Children with mind-body differences: performing disability in primary school classrooms. *Children's Geographies*, 2(2): 219–236.

Kagitcibasi, C. (1996) *Family and Human Development Across Cultures: A View from the Other Side*. London: Erlbaum.

Knapp, M., Perkins, M., Beecham, J., Dhanasiri, S. and Rustin, C. (2008) Transition pathways for young people with complex disabilities: exploring the economic consequences. *Child: Care Health and Development*, 34(4): 512–520.

Lindsay, S. and McPherson, A.C. (2012) Strategies for improving disability awareness and social inclusion of children and young people with cerebral palsy. *Child: Care Health and Development*, 38(6): 809–816.

Mitchell, W.A. (2014) Making choices about medical interventions: the experience of disabled young people with degenerative conditions. *Health Expectations*, 17(2): 254–266.

Parish, S.L. (2013) Why dismantling the safety net for children with disabilities and their families is a poor idea. *Health & Social Work*, 38(4): 195–198.

Plan International (2013) *Include Us! A Study of Disability among Plan International's Sponsored Children*. Woking: Plan International.

Scully, J.L. (2008) *Disability Bioethics: Moral Bodies, Moral Differences*. Plymouth: Rowan and Littlefield Publishers.

Shakespeare, T. (2006) *Disability Rights and Wrongs*. London: Routledge.

Shakespeare, T. and Watson, N. (2001) The social model of disability: an outdated ideology? Exploring theories and expanding methodologies. *Research in Social Science and Disability*, 2: 9–28.

Shields, N., Synnot, A.J. and Barr, M. (2012) Perceived barriers and facilitators to physical activity for children with disability: a systematic review. *British Journal of Sports Medicine*, 46(14): 989–997.

Spencer, N. and Strazdins, L. (2015) Socioeconomic disadvantage and onset of childhood chronic disabling conditions: a cohort study. *Archives of Disease in Childhood*, 100(4): 317–322.

Thomas, C. (2004a) How is disability understood? An examination of sociological approaches. *Disability & Society*, 19(6): 569–583.

Thomas, C. (2004b) Rescuing a social relational understanding of disability. *Scandinavian Journal of Disability Research*, 6(1): 22–36.

UNICEF (2013) *The State of the World's Children: Children with Disabilities*. New York, NY: United Nations.

UPIAS (1976) *Fundamental Principles of Disability*. London: Union of the Physically Impaired Against Segregation.

Part I
Theoretical and methodological practices

1 Theorising disabled childhoods

Our book explores disabled childhood across a number of related fields. These reflect the overlapping importance of the formal institutions that are present in disabled children and young people's lives, and the everyday interactions that inform their emerging sense of identity. To do so we work across a number of conceptual frameworks. Whilst these offer much to understanding childhood disability, on their own they do not sufficiently capture the range of social practices, structures, localities and relationships that inform how disabled children and young people make sense of their world and find ways through it. The arguments that have developed within disability studies are strong influences on our work, and are found across the book. What we do here is lay out what we bring from other research approaches, which can bring greater depth and complexity to our understandings of disabled childhoods. We begin by discussing some of the key ideas of childhood studies and how they can be used to think about disability (which is something they do not do); we then highlight how childhood studies writers have traced the emergence of monitoring practices regarding children in the health, educational and welfare institutions of the Global North. In the next part, we will explore the value of bringing ideas from embodiment studies into our account, and then finish by linking our work to ideas from within social studies of technology. Together, these approaches enable us to engage with the ways in which the material and the discursive come together within relational networks of meaning and practice in the multiple settings of disabled childhoods.

Childhood studies

Jenks (1996: 2) asks 'In what ways can we possibly begin to make sense of children'? This question remains at the centre of childhood studies, but with remarkably little attention given to disabled children and young people, a gap Moran-Ellis (2010) has acknowledged in her review of sociology of childhood in the UK. A quick, and granted unscientific, survey of indexes of key childhood studies texts highlights a remarkable absence of disability. For example, the recent and high profile compilation, *The Palgrave Handbook of Childhood Studies* (Qvortrup *et al.*, 2009) does not include disability in the index, although it does have two references to illness. In contrast, disability in childhood has been given significantly more attention within disability studies (Connors and Stalker, 2007; Runswick-Cole and Curran, 2013; Traustadóttir *et al.*, 2015; Watson, 2012). Here can be found an important range of literature and research exploring the historical institutionalisation of disabled children and young people; the abuses they have experienced in such institutions and other walks of life; their exclusion from society via segregation; and their gradual (and faltering) greater presence in society via policies and advocacy for social integration in areas such as education. However, the relative disinterest in childhood studies is peculiar and important. It not only means that aspects of disabled children and young people's lives are under-considered, it also means that the purpose of childhood studies is left unachieved. Studying disabled childhoods is not just about what this uncovers about disability, it is also about what it says more broadly about childhood and adolescence. In particular, we would argue that studying disability draws into the open the institutional formation of norms of childhood that affect all children and young people. The importance of focusing on a category of children and young people who are framed as incapable of being 'normal' lies, at least in part, in uncovering how their position as outsiders to childhood and adolescence plays a vital role in privileging those who are within it.

Childhood studies has at its roots a desire to move beyond the hierarchical and linear thinking of developmental psychology – a discipline which has for a long time dominated academic debates and understandings of childhood (Burman, 1994). While more willing to accept cultural variation than it is sometimes recognised for (Rogoff, 2003; Vygotski, 1929), developmental psychology nevertheless prioritises a way of studying children and young people's lives which concentrates on them as individuals – outside of history and context – learning about and adapting to the world around them. It also positions the academic interest as focused on how they develop towards adulthood – what Lee (2001) argues is a focus on children as *becomings* rather than *beings* and which Turmel (2008: 19) summarises as an interest in children as 'nothing more than a human form maturing towards adulthood'.

Developmental psychology has never fully escaped implicit, and at times explicit, hierarchies of what kinds of children and young people, and what kinds of behavioural traits, are best; not so much for the child or young person but for social order and cohesion. A strong element informing that hierarchy is the notion of the 'well adjusted' child or young person who has acquired the social skills that ensure she is able to fit in and engage with others. The problem with this hierarchy becomes obvious in the context of disability: if the goal of understanding development is to ensure that the right environment is created for the child to move towards successful adulthood, then disability is always already in deficit. It is always going to be harder to make up for that lack and repair the child to the path that should be the goal. Childhood studies asserts that children and young people are not just 'nominal ciphers' (Jenks, 1996: 10) developing towards particular ideals of adulthood, instead they are already present in the

world as people who shape it. The interest in childhood moves away from identifying how to raise the right kinds of children and young people towards highlighting the confinement contained within prescriptive accounts and measures of
the good child and child environment (James *et al.*, 1998; James and Prout,
1997). Challenging that confinement involves a deeper understanding of the
lives of children from their perspective.

To develop this deeper understanding of children and young people's lives,
childhood studies operates through two interrelated conceptual and methodological approaches. First, it adopts a broadly social constructionist framework
that emphasises the variability of norms associated with childhood. Second, it
asserts the importance of children's participation in research about their lives
(James, 1993, 2007). If children are active in creating their worlds, then it is
imperative to speak with them in order to understand how they do so (Prout,
2000a). The methodological aspect of childhood studies will be discussed in the
next chapter; for now we will focus on briefly laying out the constructionist
foundations to childhood studies.

From a social constructionist position, childhood is 'neither a natural state nor
a matter of age – but a basic component of personhood devised as a totality ...
childhood is a figure of life, a nomadic and mobile figure, continuously re-
emergent, outlined and moulded in a given culture' (Turmel, 2008: 32). Historical analyses have used this way of thinking to capture the dynamics involved in
producing childhood as a changing and varied social phenomena (Cunningham,
1991; Plumb, 1975). Ariès' (1962) key argument that childhood did not exist in
Western Europe before the eighteenth century remains – while critiqued on
several grounds (Archard, 2003; Pollock, 2003) – a corner stone of this form of
study. Ariès proposes that during the eighteenth century versions of childhood
emerged through (some) children's separation into different spaces within the
home and education, the development of styles of clothing unique to children,
the emergence of cultural materials (toys, literature, music) designed specifically
for them, and the appearance of ideals of who the child was. Children were
framed as either to be protected due to their inherent vulnerability, or to have
their wildness tamed into the performance of social order. Subsequent to Ariès,
other historians and sociologists have mapped the evolving dimensions of childhood, linking changes to the social times (Gillis, 2009). Various writers have
detailed how the practices of childhood have further delineated into distinct age
brackets, as children have split into babies, infants, young children, and adolescents (a comparatively new creation). Therefore, for childhood studies, the
answer to the question 'what turns children into children?' (Honig, 2009: 64)
lies not in understanding children's developing cognitive ability and moral consciousness, but instead *in exploring the making of the institutions of childhood
and the way children live within those institutions.*

Within this social constructionist approach an important distinction is made
between the formation of the norms of *childhood* and the lives of actual children
and young people. The cultural apparatus that children and young people exist
within are informed by what they do within them. Corsaro (2005) uses the term

'*interpretive reproduction*' to capture the active participation of children and young people in shaping their lives, within institutionalised set limits to the scope of that participation:

> The term *interpretative* captures the *innovative* and *creative* aspects of children's participation in society ... children create and participate in their own unique peer cultures by creatively taking or appropriating information from the adult world to address their own peer concerns. The term *reproduction* captures the idea that children are not simply internalising society and culture, but are actively *contributing to cultural production and change*. The term also implies that children are, by their very participation in society, *constrained by the existing social structure and by societal reproduction.*
>
> (orginal emphasis, Corsaro, 2005: 18–19)

While children and young people draw from, and limitations are produced by, the structures imposed by institutions, spaces do exist within their own peer cultures where they develop their own cultural worlds. As with other social actors, children and young people interact with the norms of being that surround them, creating opportunities for both the playing out of those norms and the challenging of them (Hardman, [1973] 2001). As should be evident from Corsaro (2005), children and young people's engagement with childhood norms emerges through the interactions they have with others. Their active presence does not occur through their individual actions or intent, but through what develops in conjunction with those around them. Everyday interactions bring broader norms and values into being, and enable the translation of those norms and values into local contexts.

Acknowledging children and young people's active presence in constructing childhood leads to two important implications. First, children and young people are important actors, through the relationships they are part of, in changes in and resistances to institutional norms. In looking at their everyday active presence in their social worlds, an important aim is to capture ways in which they provide alternative imaginaries to the dominant norms that seek to circumscribe their possibilities (Burke, 2012; Goodley and Runswick-Cole, 2010; Holt, 2004). Second, it also involves acknowledging that they can be participants in shaping the inequalities, hierarchies and exclusionary processes within the spaces they inhabit. The inequalities and exclusions children and young people experience are not just a product of the top-down imposition of normalising and marginalising norms of childhood; they are also a product of their enactment of them. It is important in studying disabled childhoods to also capture children and young people's participation in generating the boundaries that are our central concern: *the boundaries between those judged as acceptable and those framed as the other for being outside the norms of that location.*

Already it should be clear that examining the interrelationship between institutionally-produced norms of childhood and the intricacies of children's lives is more productive of understanding disability than developmental psychology.

First, the measures and criteria of developmental psychology are reframed as social constructs, linked to institutional visions of what a future successful adult citizen looks like and the steps required to reach that ideal state. Second, understanding why disabled children and young people 'fail' to meet such measures no longer involves examining their individual inadequacy; instead it involves studying the inadequacies of the measures to capture different ways, styles and paces of development and ways of being both a child and an adult. Third, such measures of appropriate childhood have been, and continue to be, politically problematic for the segregation and discrimination that they enable. Residential living and segregated education for disabled children and young people was the norm in many countries, including the UK, well into the middle of the twentieth century. Such segregation was a marker of the ways in which disabled children and young people were positioned as outside of normal childhood, so could be removed from its usual pathways. The absolute seclusion of institutional segregation may have been reduced (not eliminated) in the UK and elsewhere, however, disabled children and young people are still measured against norms of development that define them as lacking, undermining the scope of integration. Finally, scrutiny of institutionalised models of child development is integral to an understanding of the disabled child or young person as a political category. The differences in capacity that disabled children and young people enact and display become disabilities through the distance between them, the norms of appropriate childhood being, and the social and material worlds built around the expectation that those present can enact those norms.

What we draw from childhood studies is a need to engage with both the institutions of childhood (Chapters 3 and 4) and the interactive social worlds of children (Chapters 5 through 7). Childhood studies has also influenced our overall focus on monitoring and surveillance within the book, as being vital to establishing and disseminating the norms and identities of disabled childhoods.

Monitoring and surveillance

Monitoring of children and young people has been a prominent theme in childhood studies, because it is a key feature of the institutions of childhood. Processes and technologies for monitoring and surveying children and young people are core elements through which ideals of childhood are policed and certain categories of children and young people placed outside it. From Ariès (1962) onwards, writers have argued that surveillance of children has developed alongside the concept of a separate and defined period of childhood. The social history of these moves point to the interplay of overlapping goals and visions of childhood in the emergence of these practices and institutions of observation in Europe and elsewhere in the eighteenth and nineteenth centuries. Industrialisation and urbanisation were key contexts, which saw the influx of large numbers of children into both the factory workplace and the overcrowded urban environment, bringing questions about their health, wellbeing, behaviour and safety (moral as well as physical) to the fore (Blackford, 2004; Cunningham, 1995;

John, 1984). The growing scope and status of medicine and public health made it possible to collect data on infant mortality, child abuse, factory injuries, housing conditions and problems such as malnutrition, which provided important statistics for social and political debates on the consequences of rapid industrial and urban development. The plight of children was used by both newspapers and charities to highlight the problems of poverty emerging in major cities. In response, across much of the Global North, a series of legal changes removed children from the workplace and placed them instead in education (Cockburn, 2013; Sealander, 2003). Alongside this, transformative public health initiatives saw advances in housing and sanitation that produced significant improvements in child mortality and morbidity (for example James (2000: 26) quotes a reduction in infant mortality in the UK from '148 per 1000 live births in 1841–1845 to 50 in 1941–1945').

As public health initiatives began to produce improvements in health outcomes for children, Turmel (2008) argues that the focus of monitoring shifted from the prevention of illness and disease to the monitoring of children against the developing standards of 'normal childhood'. It is here, in the late nineteenth century across Europe and the US, that he argues we see the growth in processes through which normal child development was established and then children monitored and measured against (Gleason, 2005; Kellmer-Pringle, 1975; Woodhead, 2009). The institutions of education, welfare and medicine were given the job of evaluating children against these developmental criteria (Markus, 1996). Parents and children became partners in this project of institutional authority, through their deference to it and participation in the range of advice on good childrearing practice (Steedman, 1995).

Over time, the regular comparison of children against criteria of successful development has become a routinised aspect of their care by both the formal institutions of education and healthcare and the informal expectations of good parenting. Paramount within this continues to be the chart – charts of weight, height, intelligence. Think of the interest, both within families and in the institutions of school and healthcare, with children's height; it represents the bringing together of monitoring with embodiment and the formation of childhood norms. From the marks on the wall that represent the growing child, to the persistence of placing rows of children in order of height, what we see are displays of the concept that by a certain age children should be a certain height. The marks on the wall and the rows of children also speak to the importance of gazing on the child and their body, as an important element of monitoring, which may include the medical gaze, but also involves multiple processes of looking by others.

Through the multiple ways in which children's progress against key indicators of development is recorded, we can think of them as living under what Foucault (1977) referred to as 'compulsory visibility'. Lupton captures the ever-present dynamic well:

> From the time an infant is born (and even before, while *in utero*) its body is the target of constant measuring and monitoring, its bodily attributes,

growth and development noted and compared against pre-established norms. Infants are expected to conform to certain 'milestones' or markers of 'age-appropriate', 'normal' development. If they do not conform to these norms, they are typically drawn into a network of expert intervention to ensure that they do not 'fall behind'.

(Lupton, 2013: 46)

The close observation of children's progress requires a template of what the path should be, which medicine, across a number of markers of physical, emotional, behavioural and cognitive ability, has provided. Programmes are geared towards a constant fascination with growth: growth in height, in weight (the right kind of weight), in speech, in analytic skill, in empathetic awareness, and so it goes on (Kelle, 2010). The processes of monitoring have defined various markers of child development. While such measures could be thought of as averages, over time they become goals and aspirations of how to improve development. That is, value begins to be associated with what is thought of as usual, turning what is normal into a norm to be sought. As it does so, what is sought are not just children who can achieve such usual markers, but who can exceed them. The internal logic is that the norm continues to rise as expectations grow of what is usual and what is admirable. As Honig (2009: 73) argues: 'A concept of possibility and an ideal of perfection are thus linked together: childhood in modernity becomes the promise of the future, the promise of better possibilities in reality'. Crucially, these better possibilities require a contrasting other to be measured against: 'In this economy of visual difference, those bodies deemed inferior become spectacles of otherness while the unmarked are sheltered in the neutral space of normalcy' (Garland-Thomson, 1997: 8). Those without shelter are encouraged to manage their difference, work to get closer to the norm; the requirement that they do so is further evidence of the ways in which they differ from others. For those outside height norms, for example, they can manage their failure through hormone treatment to grow taller, or by getting into the habit of stooping (particularly girls) in order not to look so tall.

This is why childhood studies should be interested in disability, because disabled children and young people are crucial 'others' to the continued societal validation of the right kind of children (Garland-Thomson's '*normate*' (original emphasis, 1997: 8)). As Shildrick (1999: 79) proposes 'the standard is not normal it is normative'. Therefore, while on one level norms are fictional, they are also very real in their effects through how '[i]ndividuals regulate *themselves* in relation to the norms that circulate social spaces' (original emphasis, Holt *et al.*, 2012: 2194). Such constructs of what sits within the category of the normal and the abnormal or pathological are always in relationship with each other, co-defining the meaning each exists within (Canguilhem, 1989): 'through a priori standards that are situated within culturally and historically contingent values and practice, that which counts as 'abnormal', 'disabled', or 'pathological' is constituted and continues to be re-constituted discursively' (Lester and Paulus, 2012: 260). For some children to excel, to be shaped towards perfection, requires the presence of others who do not, who provide the contrast against which perfection can be recognised. The children who make the norm, who reach the targets, are recognised through the reflection gained by also gazing on those who do not fit, whose behaviour, bodies, and histories tell different stories about society. There is always someone at the end of the row, either who is marked as too small or too tall.

Constant monitoring has the aim of identifying gaps in a child's development, which can then be acted upon via a range of different interventions – with the ethos being, the earlier the better. Spatial and temporal dynamics have developed to ensure that children and young people are under constant surveillance. From the cautious eyes of parents, to the gaze of the health visitor and paediatrician, and the disciplining look of the teacher and social worker, little aspect or moment of childhood does not fall under the scrutiny of adults and societal institutions (Symes, 2012). Such practices help breed the requirement that they exist. For example, the proliferation of baby monitoring devices encourage the perception of ever-present risk to the infant (from the vulnerability of their own bodies, or from the actions of the others around them), leading to it being seen as a sign of child neglect not to have one (Marx and Steeves, 2010; Nelson, 2008). The strategies embedded in such programmes focus on 'constraint, control, inculcation and patterning' (Jenks, 1996: 35) and emphasise the role of parents as key agents in monitoring their children (Francis, 2012; Hays, 1996). Gillis (2009) argues that contemporary children and young people of the Global North are the most monitored and controlled in history, often justified by concerns over vulnerability and the multiple threats perceived to be present in the public sphere (Postman, 1994).

Disability studies has a long term interest in the significance of these dynamics of monitoring for disabled children and young people. Disability is in many respects a category produced by the monitoring techniques which have mushroomed since the nineteenth century. Disability studies writers argue that the practices of separating children into different categories have always been associated with varied ways that children inconvenient to the goals of social order and productive citizenship can be removed or distanced from society. As norms of development have become more prescriptive and required, the more those who appear to fall away from such norms are not just seen as different, but a problem to be treated. The practices of medical categorisation that developed in the nineteenth century produced categories of children whose physical and mental failings could be both identified and then excluded from society via their placement in institutional 'care' (Davis, L.J., 1995; Stiker, 2000). Avoiding the creation of such children was also an important justification for eugenic fascination with controlling reproduction amongst particular populations. This focus on the removal of disabled children continued well into the twentieth century through the continued use of residential care and enforced sterilisation in countries such as the United States and Scandinavia. As the use of medical justifications to completely exclude people into long-term institutional settings have become less tenable, other routes have emerged to place the socially-troubling child outside of society. One route is through disabled children and young people's over-representation within the criminal justice system (Fyson and Yates, 2011). Another is through contemporary medical categories that produce categories of embodied difference as both pathological and also something that can be removed from human possibility.

Deviations from norms of childhood development are now associated with a growing number of childhood disorders recognised via various diagnostic categories. One important way differences in development become disability is through the myriad categories we now have to define such differences as outside the prized value of normality. The emergence of childhood disorders such as Attention Deficit Hyperactivity Disorder (ADHD) have led some to argue that children's actions 'are subject to monitoring through a lens of pathology in ways unique to this historical moment' (Carpenter-Song, 2009: 64). With the multiplicity of disorders come both new forms of monitoring children to place them within the different categories, alongside new strategies for treating them (Blum, 2007; Garro and Yarris, 2009). Pharmaceutical responses are becoming routine for disorders such as ADHD, which are increasingly classified as neurological rather than behavioural in origin. Another key source of contemporary classifications of children into different categories of deviance from the norm comes from genetics. Advances in genetic technologies are allowing smaller and smaller variations in our DNA to be captured. One particular focus of genetic research is linking such variations with differences in childhood development, leading to a growing list of genetic disorders being categorised in children. Genetic knowledge of this type is used both to categorise existing children into different groupings and also to monitor the growing foetus in the womb. Screening of congenital variation, and the offer of termination if variations are found, are now routine elements of contemporary pregnancy care. The latest forms of genetic technology are also leading to dreams of manipulating DNA through techniques such as prenatal genetic diagnosis (PGD) and mitochondrial donation to ensure certain categories of children are not born. From the state eugenics of the nineteenth century, through to the laissez-faire eugenics (Fitzpatrick, 2001) of contemporary genetics, categorising children into different types is a component in attempts to define the boundaries of acceptable children (Hubbard, 1997).

Monitoring of children is an important theme of this book because of its central presence in children's lives; particularly those framed by monitoring as outside the norm. The aspects of monitoring we have highlighted so far are formal techniques that primarily emerge in the institutionalised aspects of children's lives. Another aspect of monitoring is that which occurs within the everyday, within the interactions and relationships that children and young people exist within and participate in shaping. In order to explore such interactional aspects of monitoring practice, and disabled children and young people's engagement with it, we are drawing from ideas that are associated with studies of the body, which are themselves influenced by symbolic interactionism.

Embodiment in childhood and disabled childhoods

There is a current shift occurring in disability studies (not without its critics (Vehmas and Watson, 2014)) which we both welcome and, to some degree, position our work alongside. While over-simplifying things here, disability studies is associated with an approach to embodiment that considers it to be less significant than the structures within which it exists. This focus in part emerged from an important wish to remove accounts of disability from medical concerns with the functionality of the body. Instead, what has been privileged is a need to question why society makes things so difficult for those whose bodies differ from the norm. Critical disability studies has opened up that separation to scrutiny to valuable effect, by arguing that there is a need to further establish how such bodies are recognised as different from the norm in the first place, and to ask why society has been so unwilling to embrace difference (Goodley, 2013). This clearly overlaps with our interest in both the establishment of norms and the associated dis-valuing of difference. Where we differ is in how we draw the body back into accounts of the social production of disability.

Critical disability studies has emerged from writers keen to make use of ideas from within postmodern studies, critical race studies and queer perspectives to deconstruct both disability *and* impairment as discursive all the way down (Goodley, 2013). That is, that the problem is not just that society dislikes, and is poor at managing, difference in body capacity, instead the problem is with how it produces the differences in the first place. Goodley proposes that impairment is not a product of material reality:

> To talk of the 'brute facts' of impaired or normal bodies evokes a biology that has already been constructed. Regulatory norms hail subjects to assume positions.... The body is not some entity prior to signification: it has already been through a process of signification.
>
> (Goodley, 2011: 119)

Goodley's view is that impairment is not an intrinsic property of the body; instead it is produced by categories of diagnosis and labelling. The proposal is that it is impossible to relate to disabled bodies or types of disability without it being made through language and the policing functions of linguistic norms. As Garland-Thomson (1997: 6) suggests, disability is not a property of the body, it is 'a product of cultural rules and about what bodies should be or do'. Any iden-tification of a difference between bodies is productive of the making of differ-ence. To explain why society and its key institutions have built such elaborate structures to separate people into different categories of ability and disability, critical disability studies turns to psychoanalytic ideas. The arguments of Shil-drick (2012) are crucial here. For her, the societal interest in cataloguing differ-ences develops from a need to secure normativity, which is generated by a fear of all that lies outside the desired norm. The category of normality is deeply vulnerable to the frailty of the human body; such frailty is unwelcome within the modernist imaginary of progress, of 'man's' ability to conquer nature and constantly push the boundaries of his capacities. 'Non-normative embodiment' is rejected out of a realisation that flawed bodies are the normal state of affairs – we all leak, stumble and ultimately die (Shildrick, 1997).

We sympathise with such arguments and concerns: it is vital to explore the processes of inscribing meaning onto bodies that occur through cultural negotiation and processes of identity construction and regulation. We clearly share critical disability studies' concern with how institutions such as medicine create the many categories of disability. The societal exclusion of disabled children and young people can be associated with the discomfort felt at both a personal and institutional level with those who appear unable to fit the templates provided by child development. They are 'icons of bodily vulnerability' (Garland-Thomson, 1997: 42) to be positioned outside acceptable humanity. The ways in which such children fail to comply with the medical and societal dreams of continuing to make the human condition 'better' encourages the preoccupation with seeking to fix them. However, where we move away from critical disability studies is to argue that it does not seem feasible that either the edifices of institutional power, or the lived experience of having a body differently abled than the norm, are not influenced by the body itself. In their accounts, much happens to the body but the body itself appears inert, shaped into something by modernist fantasies and cultural tropes. Within the relational networks informing the body, the body is given little role. We think it is important to hold on to the body itself in its material, as well as representative, form – including differences in the ways in which different bodies function and look. While analytically separating the social or the discursive from the material or the corporeal is impossible, a focus only on the cultural or discursive leads to an impression that only they carry significance, which is problematic.

The ways in which bodies look and function are significant in informing social interactions and are fundamental in deciding how bodies and persons 'fit' within normative frameworks of understanding. As two of us have argued elsewhere (Coleman-Fountain and McLaughlin, 2013), critical disability studies, by emphasising the cultural processes that give meaning to the body without keeping hold of its materiality, miss three important aspects of how those meanings become possible and maintained. First, some forms of bodily difference are easier to frame as particular impairments than others (Mol, 2002). Mobility problems are associated with legs or arms that inhibit movement; sight issues with eyes that are limited in function. These differences in function come to matter through the ways in which they interact with the world; but the difference is more than inscribed, it must cohere to that aspect of the body. Second, holding on to the body allows us to explore cultural hierarchies of meaning and stigma that are inscribed in, and to, different kinds of bodily difference. Different kinds of impairment lead to different levels of prejudice because of the different effects they have on how the body looks. There is a long history of associations between unusual physical features and evil (Russo, 1995; Shildrick, 2002). But it is not any bodily difference that gets equated with such folk devils. How such readings become ascribed to particular bodies and not others is an important aspect in the production of hierarchies of prejudice towards specific kinds of impairment. This occurs as much in childhood as adulthood, where the development of cultures of childhood by children and by others, are worked through hierarchies of embodiment, including disability. The third reason for keeping hold of the body is to retain an interest in what people do with their bodies as part of their participation in social interaction and the development and maintenance of a self. On a face-to-face level, it seems reasonable to acknowledge that there are forms of limitation in what the body can do that can make interaction at least more tricky when contrasted with what we perceive others to be able to do or not do. In order to retain the significance of the body as present and significant within the monitoring dynamics that revolve around disabled children and young people we turn to embodiment studies and symbolic interactionism. The value of these approaches is two-fold. First, they give greater emphasis to the role of social interaction to the relational production of disability (Kelly and Field, 1996; Vannini and Waskul, 2006). Second, the focus on interaction helps us understand why certain cultural tropes productive of disability become fixed; it is their regular presence in interaction, in what people do and say, which enables them to adhere to the social fabric of society and the embodied identities of individuals (Shilling, 1997, 1999).

Symbolic interactionism is often drawn into sociological accounts of embodiment; its value is seen in the way in which it captures the significance of everyday interactions in shaping social position and identity (Blumer, 1969). The body is drawn into its accounts through thinking of such interactions as phenomenological (Denzin, 1984; Monaghan, 2006; Waskul and Vannini, 2006). That is, a 'lived experience' within the 'perceptual, embodied world' (Jay, 2005: 283). It thus allows for an appreciation of how the ways in which we live in the world are deeply shaped by the bodies we have and our subjective, tactile experience of those bodies (Denzin, 1992). Meaning and selfhood is constructed through our embodied interactions with the social worlds that we inhabit, including the objects, technologies, social contexts and physical spaces that make up those worlds. One benefit of stressing the phenomenological aspects of interactionism is that it emphasises the emotional 'flesh and blood' of embodied interaction (Monaghan, 2006) and with that the practical accomplishments of body-subjects in their social and physical environments. Bodies do not exist as *inert* physical objects; rather they are lived, mobilised and enacted by individuals who have and are those bodies (Crossley, 2001; Vannini, 2006).

Disability has been a long-term interest in accounts of embodied interaction (Acton and Hird, 2004; Becker, 1963). Writers have explored how it 'troubles' norms of social encounters – Davis (1961) for example argued it produced 'sticky encounters'. Scully (2010) draws on symbolic interactionism to highlight the additional work that disabled people do to both interact in ways 'normal' people can relate to, and also to hide the effort involved in doing so:

> This 'dealing with,' which entails controlling one's self-presentation, identifying what the other person needs to know or wants to feel, evaluating

which strategies are needed and implementing them, producing the required responses in turn, and so on, costs significant physical and psychological energy.

(Scully, 2010: 31)

One area where symbolic interactionist work has been used in particular is exploring the stigma that is experienced not just by the disabled person, but also by those associated with them. A range of studies have used notions such as courtesy stigma to explore the lives of the families of disabled children, both to consider the work families do to protect their child from stigma in the public sphere, but also the stigma they experience because of their association with their disabled child (Farrugia, 2009; Francis, 2012; Green, 2003). This work also highlights how disabled children and young people are active agents within these interactions, labouring to pass as normal within their families and within the broader social world. Disabled children work to 'repair the fabric of the relation so that it can continue' (Garland-Thomson, 1997: 13). While at other times they also resist such social requirements for acceptance via normality (Holt, 2004). Incorporating disabled children and young people's active presence in the stigma dynamics that families experience is important to guard against research on families being about the effect of a disabled child on the broader family, rather than about the disabled child or young person's experiences of family life and their influence on shaping family life (McLaughlin, 2012).

In advocating bringing interactionism into an account of disability, it is right to acknowledge the critiques of it by disability studies scholars (Abberley, 1993; Oliver, 1990; Wendell, 1996) and others (Dennis and Martin, 2005). In particular, it has been challenged for its politically naïve understandings of the social and material contexts which inform the interactions it studies. The overall suspicion is that interactionists are oblivious to macro-structural issues due to their privileging of micro-relations that constitute 'subjective' everyday life. Nevertheless, we want to suggest that bringing symbolic interactionism, embodiment and disability in childhood together can be useful if care is taken to remain alert to questions of power and structuring conditions. Drawing these understandings of embodiment and disability into our focus on childhood allows us to acknowledge that material dynamics are important contexts for framing the meanings children and others develop around bodies, particularly those that appear different from the norms established through institutional spaces and monitoring practices (Prout, 2000b). It highlights that studying the signficance of the multiple sites of monitoring of children requires a consideration of embodiment to include what is enacted as well as what is inscribed. This allows us to examine the considerable disciplinary power enacted on the developing body, and also the opportunities that emerge for embodied resistance (Fingerson, 2009; Simpson, 2000). Such an approach 'takes account of both the materiality and experiential subjectivity of the body in the same moment that it also acknowledges the body as an objectified entity within the social world' (James, 2000: 26). Taking such ideas into the concerns of this book generates questions about:

how do particular kinds of embodiment get framed as different, by whom and in what contexts, and what are the implications of those framings?

An important component to disabled children and young people's everyday interactions is technology. Like all young people, technology is a very visible component to disabled children and young people's embodied interaction with their social worlds. Technology can also be more visible in disabled young people's lives through its role in supporting therapy, communication and everyday living (and surviving). We decided it was therefore important that we draw in theoretical work on technology and, due to our interest in monitoring and embodied materiality, we turned to social studies of technology (Latour, 1992; Law, 1991).

Social studies of technology

There are several reasons why we have given technology a particular emphasis in the book. First, it is impossible to think about and explore dynamics of monitoring and surveillance without thinking through the technologies which make such dynamics possible. Without the baby monitor, the CCTV, the weight scales, or the genetic screening test, the objectives of monitoring could not occur. Indeed it is through, as we will discuss, the possibilities for surveillance generated via these technologies that specific goals to monitor are produced. Second, as noted above, technologies are important in all children and young people's lives, but are particularly so for disabled children and young people. Finally, from within sociological work examining the significance of technology within social life, we have found valuable ideas for pursuing our interest in embodied relationality.

We include social studies of technology in our conceptual framework because of the help it provides in considering the significance of the networks disabled children and young people are located within, for the forms of regulation they experience and their possibilities for agency (Moser, 2006). Such work can help us understand the significance of a range of technologies in the formation of networks that stabilise certain social norms and ways of doing things. The range of approach and conceptualisation within social studies of technology is far broader than we can do justice to here; of particular interest to us is work that seeks to conceptualise the relational networks that form between technologies and people and others (Callon, 1986; Galis, 2011; Latour, 1996). Technology's influence in social relations is said to develop within the networks it is both part of and helps facilitate. In such accounts, both technology and humans actors are positioned in networks of technical and social relations. Callon (1991: 133) defines a network as 'a coordinated set of heterogeneous actors which interact more or less successfully to develop, produce, distribute and diffuse methods for generating goods and services'. Actors (human and non-human) form a set of practices, shared language and common meanings for each other; while the technical components of the network help keep it together. Various aspects of the operation of the network are relative – the product of the network itself. Latour (1991: 110) argues: 'Power is not a property of any one of those elements but of a chain'. A key element of network formation is the translation of different interpretations into a stable set of meanings for the network and its components. The actors in the network align themselves to what Akrich (1992) has referred to as scripts that produce frameworks of action and which link current translations to prior existing frameworks. Therefore, within such accounts, the material and the discursive come together to normalise particular ways of doing things and being. The 'other' is the subject outside of the network who falls outside due to their inability to follow the script or interact in the way expected by the network (Star, 1991).

There are a variety of ways in which ideas about networks and technologies can be drawn in to exploring disabled children and young people's lives. First, it is useful to think of disabled child embodiment as socially positioned within a range of technologically-mediated networks. While we can think of all bodies as within networks (Manning, 2009) – bodies 'cannot be separated from the spaces, objects, and other bodies with which they interact' (Lupton, 2013: 38) – such dynamics are particularly vivid in childhood. In childhood – particularly early childhood and disabled childhood – the visibility of the child's developing body and the role of others in defining it, bring the relationality of networks to the fore (Gottlieb, 2004; Lee and Motzkau, 2011). Brownlie and Sheach Leith (2011: 199) propose that 'babies are positioned at the centre of a network of actors, organisations and material practices'. The younger and/or more different the child's body, the more significant the presence of others in shaping how their body interacts with the world (Mayall, 1996) and the more they are read as bodies for others to interpret and define. Therefore 'the infant's body should be viewed, not as a container for the self, but as the site of *relationality*, the place where the self, others and the world 'out there' intermingle' (original emphasis, Brownlie and Sheach Leith, 2011: 202). Lupton (2013: 39) refers to this as 'inter-embodiment' in order to highlight how 'apparently individuated and autonomous bodies are actually experienced at the phenomenological level as intertwined'. For disabled children and young people it is possible that the additional level of scrutiny and support they receive, particularly from medicine, education and social services, may place them in particular relational dynamics that emphasise their differences from others, particularly differences that emphasise lack and deficiency (Holt *et al.*, 2012).

The second way a concern with technology is useful is the way examining it can enable us to explore its mediating role in the formation of identities of children and young people and how others engage with those identities (Place, 2000). Nelson (2008: 530) has argued that baby monitors in the home also generate a technologically-mediated relationship between parent and child, where the good parent is skilled in learning to read the sounds of the monitor, rather than the child as they 'learn to interpret their children's needs through the medium of the flashing lights'. As Prout (2000b: 13) argues, this takes us away from discussing the relationship between technology and society, to a more nuanced interest in 'the dense, networked heterogeneity that is social life'.

This positions the devices of monitoring children as being within 'a network of relationships that inherently consist of both human and non-human entities, treated symmetrically at the analytic level' (Turmel, 2008: 47). The devices that categorise weight, the developmental milestones that evaluate the adequacy of a child's progress, produce a version of the child's body that is influential in forming the boundaries between normal and abnormal, disabled and nondisabled, child and other, which have a role in shaping actual bodies as they are altered to match or work towards such norms. However, such processes of body management and modification do not occur through technologies themselves, instead it is the relational networks that make their effects possible and challengeable. What follows as a question is: *how are relations with technologies part of the production of disabled identities for children with different bodies, in particular those technologies that monitor and classify?*

Third, such analyses combine an interest in how material practice solidifies certain ways of doing things and beings that are productive of conformity and regulation, with an equal awareness of how material practice can also be a site of resistance and challenge to such regulatory dynamics. For example, Prout (2000b: 2) suggests that children emerge as 'hybrid entities' within the interwoven relationship they have with the range of material objects they and others use, providing opportunities to perform alternative ways of doing things and being a child. Turmel (2008: 34) positions childhood agency as a varied product of networks of things, practices, people and policies; that is, as a 'distributed network of subjects, bodies, materials, texts and technologies'. Agency in such a way of thinking becomes 'less an essential attribute of children and more an effect of the connections made between a heterogeneous array of materials, including bodies, representations and technologies' (Prout, 2000b: 2). It is within relational networks involving others, including technology, that opportunities for resistance to the monitoring properties of norms are most likely to occur. Through how people interact with each other in ways outside of the normal, for example making use of technologies to create new modes of communication and identity, practices are glimpsed that 'expand the norms of which lives are liveable' (Holt *et al.*, 2012: 2202).

Conclusion

From across the range of ideas we have discussed here, what is visible are a series of entanglements that are productive of shaping childhoods, which combine monitoring with care, development with prescription, norms with hierarchies. These entanglements occur through a combination of material and discursive practices that may be envisioned at the institutional level, but are made significant within the everyday worlds of disabled children and young people. We bring institutions and the everyday world of relationships together because of the interrelationship between them. We can identify how norms around disability, childhood, acceptability, the good current and future citizen, and the proper family that are generated by institutions inform the interactions of daily life. While at other moments, different ways we might interact, use technologies, or tell stories of ourselves, may provide opportunities to reject or refute such norms and offer opportunities to be different. In the actions and perspectives of disabled children and young people and those around them, we want to consider ways in which they may provide both testimony to the harms of marginalisation and also the possibilities that things could be different for all children and adults.

References

Abberley, P. (1993) Disabled people and 'normality.' In J. Swain, V. Finkelstein, S. French and M. Oliver (eds), *Disabling Barriers – Enabling Environments*. pp. 107–115. London: Sage.

Acton, C. and Hird, M. (2004) Towards a sociology of stammering. *Sociology*, 38(3): 495–513.

Akrich, M. (1992) The de-scription of technical objects. In W.E. Bijker and J. Law (eds), *Shaping Technology/Building Society: Studies in Sociotechnical Change*. pp. 225–224. Cambridge, MA: MIT Press.

Archard, D. (2003) *Children, Family and the State*. Aldershot: Ashgate.

Ariès, P. (1962) *Centuries of Childhood*. London: Jonathan Cape.

Becker, H.S. (1963) *Outsiders: Studies in the Sociology of Deviance*. New York, NY: The Free Press.

Blackford, H. (2004) Playground panopticism – ring-around-the-children, a pocketful of women. *Childhood*, 11(2): 227–249.

Blum, L.M. (2007) Mother-blame in the Prozac nation – raising kids with invisible disabilities. *Gender & Society*, 21(2): 202–226.

Blumer, H. (1969) *Symbolic Interactionism: Perspective and Method*. Englewood Cliffs, NJ: Prentice-Hall.

Brownlie, J. and Sheach Leith, V.M. (2011) Social bundles: thinking through the infant body. *Childhood*, 18(2): 196–210.

Burke, J. (2012) 'Some kids climb up; some kids climb down': culturally constructed play-worlds of children with impairments. *Disability & Society*, 27(7): 965–981.

Burman, E. (1994) *Deconstructing Developmental Psychology*. London: Routledge.

Callon, M. (1986) The sociology of an actor-network: the case of the electric vehicle. In M. Callon, J. Law and H. Rip (eds), *Mapping the Dynamics of Science and Technology: Sociology of Science in the Real World*. pp. 19–34. Basingstoke: Macmillan.

Callon, M. (1991) Techno-economic networks and irreversibility. In J. Law (ed.), *The Sociology of Monsters*. pp. 132–161. London: Routledge.

Canguilhem, G. (1989) *The Normal and the Pathological*. New York, NY: Zone Books.

Carpenter-Song, E. (2009) Caught in the psychiatric net: meanings and experiences of ADHD, pediatric bipolar disorder and mental health treatment among a diverse group of families in the United States. *Culture, Medicine and Psychiatry*, 33(1): 61–85.

Cockburn, T. (2013) *Rethinking Children's Citizenship*. Basingstoke: Palgrave Macmillan.

Coleman-Fountain, E. and McLaughlin, J. (2013) The interactions of disability and impairment. *Social Theory & Health*, 11(2): 133–150.

Connors, C. and Stalker, K. (2007) Children's experiences of disability: pointers to a social model of childhood disability. *Disability & Society*, 22(1): 19–33.

Corsaro, W.A. (2005) *The Sociology of Childhood*. Thousand Oaks, CA: Pine Forge Press.

Crossley, N. (2001) *The Social Body: Habit, Identity and Desire*. London: Sage.

Cunningham, H. (1991) *The Children of the Poor: Representations of Childhood since the Seventeenth Century*. Oxford: Blackwell.

Cunningham, H. (1995) *Children and Childhood in Western Society since 1500*. London: Longman.

Davis, F. (1961) Deviance disavowal: the management of strained interaction by the visually handicapped. *Social Problems*, 9: 120–132.

Davis, L.J. (1995) *Enforcing Normalcy: Disability, Deafness and the Body*. London: Verso.

Dennis, A. and Martin, P.J. (2005) Symbolic interactionism and the concept of power. *British Journal of Sociology*, 56(2): 191–213.

Denzin, N. (1984) *On Understanding Emotion*. San Francisco, CA: Jossey-Bass.

Denzin, N. (1992) *Symbolic Interactionism and Cultural Studies: The Politics of Interpretation*. Oxford: Blackwell.

Farrugia, D. (2009) Exploring stigma: medical knowledge and the stigmatisation of parents of children diagnosed with autism spectrum disorder. *Sociology of Health & Illness*, 31(7): 1011–1027.

Fingerson, L. (2009) Children's bodies. In J. Qvortrup, W.A. Corsaro and M.-S. Honig (eds), *The Palgrave Handbook of Childhood Studies*. pp. 217–227. Basingstoke: Palgrave.

Fitzpatrick, T. (2001) Before the cradle: new genetics, biopolicy and regulated eugenics. *Journal of Social Policy*, 30: 589–612.

Foucault, M. (1977) *Discipline and Punish: The Birth of the Prison*. New York, NY: Vintage Books.

Francis, A. (2012) Stigma in an era of medicalisation and anxious parenting: how proximity and culpability shape middle-class parents' experiences of disgrace. *Sociology of Health & Illness*, 34(6): 927–942.

Fyson, R. and Yates, J. (2011) Anti-social behaviour orders and young people with learning disabilities. *Critical Social Policy*, 31(1): 102–125.

Galis, V. (2011) Enacting disability: how can science and technology studies inform disability studies? *Disability & Society*, 26(7): 825–838.

Garland-Thomson, R. (1997) *Extraordinary Bodies: Figuring Physical Disability in American Culture and Literature*. New York, NY: New York University Press.

Garro, L.C. and Yarris, K.E. (2009) 'A massive long way': interconnecting histories, a 'special child', ADHD and everyday family life. *Culture, Medicine and Psychiatry*, 33: 559–607.

Gillis, J.R. (2009) Transitions to modernity. In J. Qvortrup, W.A. Corsaro and M.-S. Honig (eds), *The Palgrave Handbook of Childhood Studies*. pp. 114–126. Basingstoke: Palgrave Macmillan.

Gleason, M. (2005) From 'disgraceful carelessness' to 'intelligent precaution': accidents and the public child in English Canada, 1900–1950. *Journal of Family History*, 30(2): 230–241.

Goodley, D. (2011) *Disability Studies*. London: Sage.

Goodley, D. (2013) Dis/entangling critical disability studies. *Disability & Society*, 28(5): 631–644.

Goodley, D. and Runswick-Cole, K. (2010) Emancipating play: dis/abled children, development and deconstruction. *Disability & Society*, 25(4): 499–512.

Gottlieb, A. (2004) *The Afterlife Is Where We Come From: The Culture of Infancy in West Africa*. London and Chicago, IL: The University of Chicago Press.

Green, S.E. (2003) 'What do you mean "what's wrong with her?"': stigma and the lives of families of children with disabilities. *Social Science & Medicine*, 57: 1361–1374.

Hardman, C. ([1973] 2001) Can there be an Anthropology of Children? *Childhood*, 8(4): 501–517.

Hays, S. (1996) *The Cultural Contradictions of Motherhood*. London and New Haven, CT: Yale University Press.

Holt, L. (2004) Children with mind-body differences: performing disability in primary school classrooms. *Children's Geographies*, 2(2): 219–236.

Holt, L., Lea, J. and Bowlby, S. (2012) Special units for young people on the autistic spectrum in mainstream schools: sites of normalisation, abnormalisation, inclusion, and exclusion. *Environment and Planning A*, 44: 2191–2206.

Honig, M.-S. (2009) How is the child constituted in childhood studies? In J. Qvortrup, W.A. Corsaro and M.-S. Honig (eds), *The Palgrave Handbook of Childhood Studies*. pp. 62–77. Basingstoke: Palgrave Macmillan.

Hubbard, R. (1997) Abortion and disability: who should and who should not inhabit the world? In L.J. Davis (ed.), *The Disability Studies Reader*. pp. 187–200. London: Routledge.

James, A. (1993) *Childhood Identities: Self and Social Relationships*. Edinburgh: Edinburgh University Press.

James, A. (2000) Embodied being(s): understanding the self and the body in childhood. In A. Prout (ed.), *The Body, Childhood and Society*. pp. 19–37. Basingstoke: Palgrave.

James, A. (2007) Giving voice to children's voices: practices and problems, pitfalls and potentials. *American Anthropologist*, 109(2): 261–272.

James, A. and Prout, A. (eds) (1997) *Constructing and Reconstructing Childhood: Contemporary Issues in the Sociological Study of Childhood*. London: Routledge Falmer.

James, A., Jenks, C. and Prout, A. (1998) *Theorizing Childhood*. Cambridge: Polity Press.

Jay, M. (2005) *Songs of Experience: Modern American and European Variations on a Universal Theme*. Berkeley, CA: University of California Press.

Jenks, C. (1996) *Childhood*. London: Routledge.

John, A. (1984) *By the Sweat of Their Brow: Women Workers at Victorian Coal Mines*. London: Routledge and Kegan Paul.

Kelle, H. (2010) 'Age-appropriate development' as a measure and a norm: an ethnographic study of the practical anthropology of routine paediatric check-ups. *Childhood*, 17(1): 9–25.

Kellmer-Pringle, M. (1975) *The Needs of Children*. London: Hutchinson.

Kelly, M.P. and Field, D. (1996) Medical sociology, chronic illness and the body. *Sociology of Health & Illness*, 18(2): 241–257.

Latour, B. (1991) Technology is society made durable. In J. Law (ed.), *The Sociology of Monsters*. pp. 103–131. London: Routledge.

Latour, B. (1992) Where are the missing masses? The sociology of a few mundane artifacts. In W. Bijker and J. Law (eds), *Shaping Technology/Building Society*. pp. 20–43. Cambridge, MA: MIT Press.

Latour, B. (1996) *Aramis, or the Love of Technology*. Cambridge, MA: Harvard University Press.

Law, J. (ed.) (1991) *A Sociology of Monsters: Essays on Power, Technology and Domination*. London and New York, NY: Routledge.

Lee, N. (2001) *Childhood and Society*. Buckingham: Open University Press.

Lee, N. and Motzkau, J.F. (2011) Navigating the bio-politics of childhood. *Childhood*, 18(1): 7–19.

Lester, J.N. and Paulus, T.M. (2012) Performative acts of autism. *Discourse & Society*, 23(3): 259–273.

Lupton, D. (2013) Infant embodiment and inter-embodiment: a review of sociocultural perspectives. *Childhood*, 20(1): 37–50.

Manning, E. (2009) What if it didn't all begin and end with containment? Toward a leaky sense of self. *Body & Society*, 15(3): 33–45.

Markus, T.A. (1996) Early nineteenth century school space and ideology. *Paedagogica Historica*, 32(1): 9–50.

Marx, G. and Steeves, V. (2010) From the beginning: children as subjects and agents of surveillance. *Surveillance and Society*, 7(3/4): 192–230.

Mayall, B. (1996) *Children, Health and the Social Order*. Buckingham: Open University Press.

McLaughlin, J. (2012) Understanding disabled families: replacing tales of burden with ties of interdependency. In N. Watson, C. Thomas and A. Roulstone (eds), *Routledge Companion to Disability Studies*. pp. 402–413. London: Routledge.

Mol, A. (2002) *The Body Multiple: Ontology in Medical Practice*. Durham, NC: Duke University Press.

Monaghan, L.F. (2006) Corporeal indeterminacy: the value of embodied, interpretive sociology. In D.D. Waskul and P. Vannini (eds), *Body/Embodiment: Symbolic Interactionism and the Sociology of the Body*. pp. 125–140. Aldershot: Ashgate.

Moran-Ellis, J. (2010) Reflections on the sociology of childhood in the UK. *Current Sociology*, 58(2): 186–205.

Moser, I. (2006) Disability and the promises of technology: technology, subjectivity and embodiment within an order of the normal. *Information, Communication & Society*, 9(3): 373–395.

Nelson, M.K. (2008) Watching children – describing the use of baby monitors on www. Epinions.com *Journal of Family Issues*, 29(4): 516–538.

Oliver, M. (1990) *The Politics of Disablement*. Basingstoke: Macmillan.

Place, B. (2000) Constructing the bodies of critically ill children: an ethnography of intensive care. In A. Prout (ed.), *The Body, Childhood and Society*. pp. 172–194. Basingstoke: Palgrave.

Plumb, J.H. (1975) The new world of children in eighteenth century England. *Past and Present*, 67: 64–93.

Pollock, L. (2003) *Forgotten Children: Parent-Child Relations from 1500 to 1900*. Cambridge: Cambridge University Press.

Postman, N. (1994) *The Disappearance of Childhood*. New York, NY: Vintage Press.

Prout, A. (2000a) Children's participation: control and self-realisation in British late modernity. *Children & Society*, 14(4): 304–315.

Prout, A. (2000b) Childhood bodies: construction, agency and hybridity. In A. Prout (ed.), *The Body, Childhood and Society*. pp. 1–18. Basingstoke: Palgrave.

Qvortrup, J., Corsaro, W.A. and Honig, M.-S. (eds) (2009) *The Palgrave Handbook of Childhood Studies*. Basingstoke: Palgrave Macmillan.

Rogoff, B. (2003) *The Cultural Nature of Human Development*. Oxford: Oxford University Press.

Runswick-Cole, K. and Curran, T. (eds) (2013) *Disabled Children's Childhood Studies: Critical Approaches in a Global Context*. Basingstoke: Palgrave Macmillan.

Russo, M. (1995) *The Female Grotesque: Risk, Excess and Modernity*. London: Routledge.

Scully, J.L. (2010) Hidden labor: disabled/nondisabled encounters, agency and autonomy. *International Journal of Feminist Approaches to Bioethics*, 3(2): 25–42.

Sealander, J. (2003) *The Failed Century of the Child*. Cambridge: Cambridge University Press.

Shildrick, M. (1997) *Leaky Bodies and Boundaries: Feminism, Postmodernism and (Bio) Ethics*. London: Routledge.

Shildrick, M. (1999) The body which is not one: dealing with differences. *Body & Society*, 5(2–3): 77–92.

Shildrick, M. (2002) *Embodying the Monster: Encounters with the Vulnerable Self*. London: Sage.

Shildrick, M. (2012) Critical disability studies: rethinking the conventions for the age of postmodernity. In N. Watson, A. Roulstone and C. Thomas (eds), *Routledge Handbook of Disability Studies*. pp. 30–41. London: Routledge.

Shilling, C. (1997) Emotions, embodiment and the sensation of society. *Sociological Review*, 45(2): 195–219.

Shilling, C. (1999) Towards an embodied understanding of the structure/agency relationship. *British Journal of Sociology*, 50(4): 543–562.

Simpson, B. (2000) Regulation and resistance: children's embodiment during the primary-secondary school transition. In A. Prout (ed.), *The Body, Childhood and Society*. pp. 60–78. Basingstoke: Macmillan Press.

Star, S.L. (1991) Power, technologies and the phenomenology of conventions: on being allergic to onions. In J. Law (ed.), *A Sociology of Monsters*. pp. 26–56. London: Routledge.

Steedman, C.K. (1995) *Strange Dislocations. Childhood and the Idea of Human Interiority, 1780–1980*. London: Virago.

Stiker, H.-J. (2000) *A History of Disability*. Ann Arbor, MI: The University of Michigan Press.

Symes, C. (2012) No time on their hands: children and the narrative architecture of school diaries. *Time & Society*, 21(2): 156–174.

Traustadóttir, R., Ytterhus, B., Thóra Egilson, S. and Berg, B. (2015) *Childhood and Disability in the Nordic Countries: Being, Becoming, Belonging*. Basingstoke: Palgrave Macmillan.

Turmel, A. (2008) *A Historical Sociology of Childhood*. Cambridge: Cambridge University Press.

Vannini, P. (2006) Symbolic interaction as music: the esthetic constitution of meaning, self, and society. *Symbolic Interaction*, 29(1): 5–18.

Vannini, P. and Waskul, D.D. (2006) Body-ekstasis: socio-semiotic reflections on surpassing the dualism of body-image. In D.D. Waskul and P. Vannini (eds), *Body/Embodiment: Symbolic Interaction and the Sociology of the Body*. pp. 123–143. Aldershot: Ashgate.

Vehmas, S. and Watson, N. (2014) Moral wrongs, disadvantages, and disability: a critique of critical disability studies. *Disability & Society*, 29(4): 638–650.

Vygotski, L.S. (1929) The problem of the cultural development of the child. *Journal of Genetic Psychology*: 415–432.

Waskul, D.D. and Vannini, P. (2006) *Body/Embodiment: Symbolic Interaction and the Sociology of the Body*. Aldershot: Ashgate.

Watson, N. (2012) Theorising the lives of disabled children: how can disability theory help? *Children & Society*, 26(3): 192–202.

Wendell, S. (1996) *The Rejected Body: Feminist Philosophical Reflections on Disability*. New York, NY: Routledge.

Woodhead, M. (2009) Child development and the development of childhood. In J. Qvortrup, W.A. Corsaro and M.-S. Honig (eds), *The Palgrave Handbook of Childhood Studies*. pp. 46–61. Basingstoke: Palgrave Macmillan.

2 Methodological approaches

The research that is drawn upon across the book does not represent a body of work planned ahead to examine 'monitoring disabled children and young people'. Instead, over a decade (the first project began in 2003, the last ended in 2013), research concerns and approaches evolved and contexts changed. Various factors effected the emergence of the different projects and their research foci and design. As will become clear, while one of us (McLaughlin) was involved in all three projects, in each project the team varied, bringing different ideas, methodological expertise and theoretical resources. Below we acknowledge who participated in each project. The other two authors of this book (Clavering and Coleman-Fountain), as well as playing key roles as research associates in different aspects of the fieldwork, also continue to be involved in the development and writing of the specific ideas we are discussing here. Another factor that has shaped the changing development of the projects has been how the themes of one have influenced the themes of the next through the ideas expressed by research participants. A final aspect that has influenced the way the projects have been designed has been the involvement of a range of organisations and actors who either represent disabled children and their families, or work with them from within health and social care. The varied roles such individuals have played, whether co-investigators or advisors, have again helped inform our priorities and they have been important facilitators of multiple aspects of the projects and their dissemination to non-academic actors. Children and young people have increasingly played this role in our research partnership activities.

As will become clear in the brief summaries below, the projects have not just involved working with children and young people, indeed the first two primarily involved working directly with adults, often, but not exclusively, parents. In addition, most (but not all) of our advisors and partners have been from adult worlds, including from the worlds which we associate with dynamics of regulation and monitoring. One of the core values of contemporary work on children and young people is that it be done *with* them and increasingly be shaped *by* them (Christensen and James, 2000; Kellett, 2005). Childhood and youth studies has been central in the calls for this kind of approach and the development of research techniques said to enable children's voices to be heard. In addition, the United Nations Convention on the Rights of the Child has placed a greater emphasis on policy makers and practitioners being informed by the voices of children – including disabled children – in both their individual care and the design of policy (Franklin and Sloper, 2006; Shaw *et al.*, 2011; Todd, 2012). We can think of such calls as a challenge to the social and institutional dynamics of monitoring and regulation we are exploring in the book. Instead of being the object of scrutiny, children and young people are being called on to be chroniclers of their worlds, to provide testimony about what it is like to be positioned as such objects. Research in this understanding becomes a 'political act – it challenges ideas about who has expertise and who does not' (Save the Children, 2004: 14). There is, therefore, a need for us to explore and explain the role adults have played in our research approach and to respond to the calls for children themselves to be the authors of their own stories. We do so by supporting such calls, but also by justifying why adults can have a role in examining the themes we have been working on through our projects, and through which the theme of monitoring children became central to what we are examining here. To summarise: we do not see the adults we have worked with as being 'proxies' to gaining children and young people's perspectives. Instead they are included in our research as being important elements in the relational networks which inform young people's lives. We speak to them not as people who can provide testimony on the lives of their children, rightly this should come from children themselves, but as important actors whose own identities, social positions, and values will be influential.

The studies

Several factors are shared across all three projects.

- Each of the studies was funded by the UK's Economic and Social Research Council (ESRC) and involved multiple team members and a range of qualitative research design practices.
- The projects were all undertaken in the North of England. This influenced the projects in a number of ways. We have worked over a large geographical area, across post-industrial cities, and comparatively remote and marginalised small towns and villages still living with the effects of the decline of coal and ship building industries. Researchers often speak of the challenge of over-representation of middle class voices in research. In each of our projects we always have been able to include people from backgrounds they defined (proudly) as working class and for whom experiences of significant economic precarity were important aspects of their lives. This remained constant from before austerity hit the UK, through the period of recession that followed, and has carried on into the long term retrenchment of the welfare state and the broader economic marginalisation of the North of England in the present day. While class and social and economic marginalisation were not things we had built into our research design, they have remained important factors in the findings that have emerged.

- Each project obtained ethics approval from NHS regional ethics committees. In addition, because each included recruitment through NHS-held databases and gatekeepers, they also involved going through NHS research and development (R&D) governance structures. The R&D governance structures at times generated problems in terms of the fit between their procedures for evaluating health research practice and social research seeking to work with people in flexible and responsive ways. In particular, their regulatory protocols were heavily bureaucratic (we would say increasingly so in the lifetime of these research projects) and unresponsive to reflexive and emergent ethical practice.
- When discussing research participants we always use fictional names, however issues relating to identifiability are more substantial than not just using real names. One project (*Embodied Transitions*) has specific issues relating to the use of visual material that are discussed below.
- The projects all had advisory groups made up of actors who were researchers, practitioners in the area, support group workers and people with direct experience of the issues being examined.

Enabling Care project

The first project began in 2003 and was titled 'Professionals and Disabled Babies: Identifying Enabling Care'. Throughout the book we will refer to it as *Enabling Care*. The idea for the project emerged in discussions between McLaughlin and a colleague, Dan Goodley. McLaughlin was interested in critiques of professional knowledge and power, and feminist theories around the ethics of care, while Goodley brought an expertise in disability studies as a way to rethink the lives of families with disabled young children. Alongside Goodley (who was the project's principal investigator) and McLaughlin, the project had three research associates: Emma Clavering (who worked with McLaughlin) and Pamela Fisher and Claire Tregaskis (who worked with Goodley). Our focus was the early years of having an infant or baby diagnosed as having some form of disability, and to examine what this meant for the family in terms of looking after the child, and their experiences of doing so with the multiple medical, social and educational professionals involved in their lives. We aimed to explore how parents' understandings of themselves and the world around them changed over time, what transitions occurred within their lives, and how they articulated those changes and responded to them. The research, which took three and a half years, was based in two English regions (the North of England and the Midlands); at the centre of the fieldwork were 39 families. The research involved longitudinal narrative interviews with families done over a two-year period, observations of formal and informal care encounters, and mixed focus groups with healthcare, social care and education professionals.

The material drawn from this project in the book is that undertaken by Clavering and McLaughlin in the North of England (to explore the findings from across the study as a whole, and for a longer discussion of the methodological challenges in the project see McLaughlin *et al.* (2008)). In this arm of the study we worked with 12 families over a period of two years, undertaking 40 interviews and 25 observations. We also undertook three focus groups with professionals. The families came from a variety of social backgrounds and lived their lives in different family and caring forms. Using occupation and housing situation as a measure of class, the majority of families were living working class lives, with a small number lower middle class or middle class. In the research we did not seek to target particular conditions, this would be within a medical model we sought to distance ourselves from. Instead, the basis for a family's inclusion was that they defined their child as having specific care and support needs and that the child was within the age range used in the project. This strategy led to a variety of conditions and labels being included in the research. In the vast majority of cases the mother, in both married and single households, was the main carer for the child.

Genetic Journeys project

In the *Enabling Care* project a small number of families had a child with differences in their development that had triggered a referral to a genetics service. Discussions with the families and with a local family support group (Contact a Family North East) led us to identify this as an area that warranted further study. The families had discussed issues around the specific dynamics of their interactions with the genetic service that appeared different from other experiences, in particular that these encounters involved close examination of the child's features and body, that they took place over time, and generated lots of uncertainties over what could be found and if something was found what it meant. It also often led to the broader family, past and present, being drawn into the genetic investigations. We spoke with geneticists who indicated they were keen to know more about what it was like for children and their families to have their bodies, their family's present and past, and their genetic makeup placed under such close medical scrutiny. In discussion with a genetics service and Contact a Family North East we developed a proposal for the ESRC that was funded in 2008. The project was titled 'Kinship and Genetic Journeys: A Study of the Experiences of Families who are Referred to Paediatric Genetics' and the full team, alongside McLaughlin, was Emma Clavering (research associate), Erica Haimes (co-investigator) and Michael Wright (co-investigator). In the book we will refer to it as *Genetic Journeys*. The aim of the project was to follow families through their diagnostic 'journey' and also to explore experiences of living with or without a genetic diagnosis (at the time, around 50 per cent of children referred to a UK genetics service would not receive a definitive diagnosis, this is now changing with the advent of new diagnostic tests and technologies).

The project took place over three years, with two years spent undertaking fieldwork. It began via recruiting families with a child referred to the genetics service and through calls for participants through the local family support group. We defined family members as those who had an ongoing close relationship with the child, the boundaries of who that included was established (and at times changed) through the research process. The service we recruited through was based within one Hospital Trust, but undertook clinics across a large rural and urban region. Their referrals, usually triggered by a paediatrician, led to an initial consultation at one of the clinics. Referrals were most often addressed to parents, asking them and their child to attend the clinic. If, after an initial visual examination of the child and questions directed at the parents regarding family history, the geneticist thought there was something they could look for, then further consultations and tests would occur. This move to biochemical analyses did not always begin after the first consultation. At times, the genetic consultant would instead ask for the child to come back after six months or so, the aim being to see whether their further development, including changes in their physical appearance, would provide further 'clues' regarding which particular trait or syndrome might be affecting the child. Consultants referred to this process as 'watchful waiting'.

The methodological approach was to follow each family over time as they made their diagnostic journey, going with them into the different settings of their lives, and listening to the perspectives of multiple family actors, including parents, siblings, other significant family members and the children who had been referred. The majority of the families we worked with were recruited as the process of first referral to the genetics service was underway and we followed them through their first consultation and beyond. At this stage the child referred was very young, between two and five years old. The project also recruited a smaller group who were several years on from referral and we spoke with them to examine their experiences of living with or without a diagnosis. Fieldwork data was generated through a mix of qualitative longitudinal interviews and non-participant observation in clinical and non-clinical encounters. From the design stage, we made a very conscious decision that children themselves would be directly involved in the research. Because the study examined those living with or without a diagnosis it included children older than the infants who had been involved in the previous study. We felt it important to engage directly with these children, both those referred and their siblings, as important actors within the relational networks of family being opened up to scrutiny by the geneticists and by us. In addition, due to our engagement with childhood studies and its arguments in favour of working with children, we recognised it was important to include them as key actors in the diagnostic journey. Children who were around ten and above were approached via their families to explore whether they would like to participate. In families where we were aiming to work with the children, the first recruitment approach was via the parents, but the family only became involved if both parents and children wanted to participate. In one case a mother was very keen to be involved, but her daughter who was 13 and had been seen at various points in her life by a genetics service due to a series of problems she faced, was not. Her view was that speaking to us was another example of others (adult others) focusing on her embodied difference as the one aspect of her that was of interest. Therefore, we followed her request and withdrew from being involved with the family as a whole.

In choosing our methods for working directly with children and young people, we were influenced by the accounts of those working with children who advocate the importance of finding ways to tap into their perspectives, which escape the power and hierarchies of knowledge that can be embedded in children being interviewed by adults (discussed in more detail below). The children and young people were given the option of filling in journals with their stories, drawings and thoughts on what family and genetics meant to them. After they had spent some time with the journals, the researcher then returned to the family home to talk to them about what they were seeking to express. Alongside this direct work with children, other children's perspectives and agency did have a presence in the fieldwork. In the observations of the families with very young children being seen by the genetic service we saw ways in which the presence, perspectives and desires of the infant were playing a role in the medical encounter and in the broader family life. While these young children did not formally participate through interviews, the opportunities we had to see them within their different relational networks influenced our findings. They also influenced whether we would indeed be present in such interactions. Where the young children were only present in the research through being observed in their clinical and non-clinical encounters, consent was granted via the parents. However, before the first observation, the children, as well as the parents, met with the researcher who would be present. During this encounter a key aim was to enable the child to become familiar with the researcher. When observations then took place, if there was any indication that the presence of the researcher was unsettling the child, the observation would end.

A total of 26 families participated in the study. This included:

- 44 adults (38 parents, two aunts, three grandmothers, and one grandfather) who each undertook up to three interviews with us.
- 27 children (aged between five months and 18 years old) who we observed either in clinic consultations or in their everyday life.
- Nine children and young people who agreed to produce journals and discuss them with the researcher, five of whom had been referred to the genetics clinic, and four siblings. They were aged between nine and 18 years old.

Each of the projects has faced a number of ethical challenges and issues that go beyond what is dealt with by gaining formal ethical approval. In this project, three overlapping issues were particularly important. First, we were recruiting many of our participants from a service closely involved in their care, as well as observing some of that care. It was important during the fieldwork, and remains important in our writing up of our findings, that we do as much as we can to ensure that clinic staff cannot identify who participated in the study. To guard against this we recruited families who agreed to have consultations observed, but for whom no data would be generated in terms of observation notes and no analysis would be undertaken. This meant that service staff would not know which families observed were included in the study in terms of data and analysis. Second, the types of genetic trait being looked for in these consultations are often very rare; if those traits are named by us, and this is then linked to the knowledge that we work in the North of England, identification becomes at least theoretically possible. Because of this we do not provide information on specific diagnoses and aspects of the specific chromosomal variations found are at times altered. Finally, due to ESRC funding, it was a requirement that data from the project was submitted to a qualitative data archive that other academic researchers can access. We understand the value of doing this, but had concerns due to the sensitivity of the data and the ways in which it had been produced via close relationships between the researcher and the families, which the data would be divorced from in the archive. We decided that the journal and conversational data from the children and young people and the observation notes would not be included, only the interview material with adults. At the beginning of the study people gave or refused consent for the interviews to be included in the data archive. However, we felt it a more meaningful decision if it occurred after interviews had been done and transcripts returned (as is our standard practice). When we re-sought consent at the end of the study, several of those who had initially said yes withdrew their consent.

In the first interviews, adult participants (as individuals rather than as 'a family') were asked a range of broad demographic questions, that included what class they identified with – something which often generated rich and highly relevant data about their identity, which became important to our analysis of their accounts. What was evident from those discussions was that the majority defined themselves as working class and this identity was deeply important and meaningful to them.

Embodied Transitions project

The observational work we undertook in the *Genetics Journeys* project, particularly in the clinic consultations, drew our attention to the ways in which a child's body can become the object of scrutiny due to how it differs from norms of how children's bodies should look, function and interact with the world. Such issues had also been visible in the *Enabling Care* project when parents talked about other people's reactions to their children because of their physical and enacted differences. We became interested in examining this further, particularly from the perspective of children and young people themselves: how do they live with and through bodies seen by others as different, how does this change over time as their bodies change due to growing up, and to what degree do values of normality play a part in their embodied identities? An opportunity to explore these themes came through an invitation to develop qualitative work with disabled young people to sit alongside a large scale European comparative quantitative research programme (Study of Participation of Children with Cerebral Palsy Living in Europe, SPARCLE). SPARCLE had been working with a cohort of young people with cerebral palsy since they were children. We designed a project with the aim of working with participants in the study from the North of England and were able to obtain funding from the ESRC in 2011. The project was called 'Embodied Selves in Transition: Disabled Young Bodies', and the full team involved, alongside McLaughlin were: Edmund Coleman-Fountain (research associate), Allan Colver (co-investigator) and Patrick Olivier (co-investigator). In the book we will refer to the project as *Embodied Transitions*. In the study, which took over two years, we worked with young people who had been part of SPARCLE since their childhood, including some who had participated in qualitative interviews when they were between eight and 12 years old, alongside some other young people with cerebral palsy we recruited via a local school.

In total, 17 disabled young people participated: thirteen from SPARCLE and four from the local school. The sample included ten young men and seven young women aged between 14 and 20 at the beginning of the fieldwork. Each participant had a diagnosis of cerebral palsy and all had physical impairments that affected them in varied ways. While we did not ask the young people what they felt to be their class position, reflecting on their home's location and family context, they were from a mix of working class and middle class backgrounds, with a smaller representation of people living in precarious situations than we have had in other projects. To explore young people's perspectives on living in a body others defined as different, we wanted to draw from methods more engaging to them and which could capture embodied practices (Morrow, 2001). Our starting point was that they were 'capable, social actors' (O'Kane, 2000: 133) able to both discuss and represent their lives. The project worked through various phases, at each phase the participants could decide whether they wanted to participate. In the first phase, we undertook face-to-face narrative interviews exploring both their memories of childhood and their current embodied practices and perspectives. With those who had undertaken SPARCLE interviews as children, we shared interview extracts with them (we also obtained their consent for us to access the childhood interviews and use them in analysis). The next phase was to undertake some photographic 'tasks'. We gave them the choice of using their own photographic equipment, or equipment we would provide which was designed to be easy to use. The clear majority chose to use cameras they already owned (mostly on mobile phones) and photographs they already had. They also had the choice to share the photographs with us in a variety of ways, including via a closed Facebook group within which they would also be able to see pictures taken by other research participants, or using journals of the type we had used in the *Genetic Journeys* project. Virtually all chose journals; when we discussed their choices with them it was clear that they both enjoyed the creative and tactile experience of producing the journal, and that they preferred the security of sharing this material with the researcher they had met, rather than online with people they had not. Virtual methods are often held to be more appealing to young people, given their immersion in social media; this is just one small example of how it is better to explore with young people how they want to work, rather than assume certain techniques are more appealing to them.

In the journals, they 'curated' the photographs alongside brief explanations of what the photographs meant to them. We provided tasks, for example 'memories of childhood', or 'what you like about how you look now', to aid their photographic work, but they also could engage with the visual work in ways that meant sense to them – and several did. Similarly to the *Genetic Journeys* project, an interview was then undertaken to explore the journals or photographs taken. Interestingly, this provided a more tangible prompt into discussing memories of childhood than had looking at their SPARCLE childhood interviews. Photographs they shared of themselves in hospital, or some of the medical devices such as callipers they had worn as children, led to long discussions of what it had been like to spend significant periods of childhood in hospital, or undertaking painful medical procedures. Finally, participants were invited to participate in two workshops where, joined by digital jeweller Jayne Wallace, we explored how designing artefacts that included personal belongings could be a device for both broader discussion and the creation of representative artefacts that conveyed their perspective and which they could then wear.

Working with the photography was the area of most ethical concern in this project. We had to think through what advice to give the participants in terms of photographs they took, particularly ones in public places and ones involving others. After photographs were shared with us, we created digital copies that were saved on a secure network and returned the originals to the participants. This way the photographs, as well as the journals some had made and spent considerable time putting together, could be kept by them (the same process had been used in the *Genetic Journeys* project). Before ending our research relationship with them we went through all photographs and identified ones which we might want to use in public domains such as conferences and publications. These were sent to the participants with an explanation of how we might use them, and instructions for them to give or refuse consent for each photo to be used. Only photographs which they gave such consent for are ever publicly used by us. We designed a website at the end of the project (The Body Matters Project, http:// research.ncl.ac.uk/thebodymatters/), in consultation with the research panel discussed below. When designing the website, we decided that we could not control how images placed online might be acquired, manipulated and used, so decided not to use the images the young people had produced in that location. Instead, an artist created sketches based on their photographs.

The fieldwork processes we undertook in the project were designed with input from disabled young people. Working with local groups of disabled young people linked to ongoing activities led by local city councils on issues of disabled young people's social participation, we put together a panel who advised us on various aspects of research focus, design and dissemination. For example, the original research design was that we would provide specifically-designed digital cameras, which would enable us to explore new digital methodological practices. However, the panel recommended instead we give participants the choice to use their existing camera technologies, which they were familiar with – which the majority of participants opted to do.

This example of using a panel of disabled young people to inform research design speaks to the focus on co-production in research practice. Such involvement of young people in research design is encouraged by contemporary research on childhood. We cannot claim what we did represents the intensity of participatory practice that could legitimately be referred to as co-production, for example the panel was put together after we had funding rather than before, so did not participate in shaping research questions, and they informed our research practice, rather than participated in it. Nevertheless, as our projects have developed, and we have engaged more with children and young people themselves, we have become more influenced by the debates about how and why children and young people should be included in research practice. Our work now draws more from such approaches, while also pursuing a slightly different path, particularly the continued involvement of adults. Now we have established what we did in the different projects, we would like to spend a little time exploring the arguments around children and young people's participation in research and how it has increasingly influenced our practice, and also how we still see a value in working with adults alongside children and young people.

Children and young people's participation in research

As indicated at the beginning of this chapter, the arguments from within childhood and youth studies that children and young people can be capable social actors conscious of the world around them, linked to the emergence of children's rights on the policy and legal agenda, has led to a significant increase in research not just *about* children and young people, but in some way *by* them (Alderson, 2001; Kellett, 2010; Mason and Hood, 2010; Melton *et al.*, 2013). Such calls have led to important and valuable changes in both existing techniques for bringing children and young people into the design, practice and management of research and in new techniques for gathering and understanding their perspectives as research participants. Some have talked of a research continuum of practice (Clavering and McLaughlin, 2010), others a ladder (Hart, 1992), which document the increasing role of children and young people within research, with the ultimate goal and ideal being 'user-led' research, with the children and young people at the centre. It is an important change that research should now begin by asking how children and young people can be involved and what is the purpose of the research and that involvement: in short, whose interest does it serve?

It is now widely recognised that working with children and young people in research about their lives enhances the validity and credibility of research, drawing on the expertise they have in evaluating the world around them (Nabors, 2013; Shaw *et al.*, 2011). As Save the Children (2004: 10) have summarised 'Perhaps the principal argument for children being more actively involved in research concerning them is that it is their right. Boys and girls have the right to decide if they wish to get involved, to what degree and how'. Various children's organisations have produced 'toolkits' for developing approaches that work with children and young people, engaging with all aspects of the research process, from identifying the research question/topic, through to research practice, and on to analysis and dissemination (Save the Children, 2000). These toolkits and approaches call for an opening-up of technique to enable the adult researcher to step from their adult world into the world of children and young people. Writers talk of the need for researchers to become 'atypical adults' or to take on 'least adult roles'. The goal in doing so is to signal to children and young people that researchers are different from the adults they usually interact with, because the researcher wishes to learn *from* them, rather than impart knowledge and wisdom *on to* them. Emphasis is also given in seeking permission to enter children's worlds (Christensen, 2004; Valentine, 1999; Warming, 2011). Ethnographic approaches are seen as one way to develop the trust that enables such permission to be real and to embed the researcher in the worlds of children and young people (Warming, 2011).

While qualitative interviews are still said to have a role in research with children and young people, particularly if they are as open-ended and conversational as possible, there is recognition that on their own they may fail to step outside the power dynamic of the adult-child interaction children usually find themselves in. In response, the majority of researchers working with children now speak of the importance of multiple and flexible methods that can give children choice in what they do and which echo other ways in which children interact with the social world. Multi-method designs are said to make participation in research more interesting for children and young people by giving greater flexibility in how data is produced, and can enable different yet complementary insights into the meanings they make of their worlds (Bagnoli, 2011; Darbyshire *et al.*, 2005). Of particular interest to researchers is making use of creative approaches such as drawing, photography and storytelling as ways to connect with children's imagination (Kullman, 2012; Punch, 2002). Such approaches have been taken up particularly within work with disabled children and young people. Disabled childhoods researchers point out that the interview process can be problematic for disabled children and young people who may face limitations in traditional or mainstream forms of cognition and communication (Sutherland and Young, 2014). Another way researchers seek to open up the research process to work more engagingly with children and young people is to involve children and young people as 'co-researchers'; that is, to draw from participatory research approaches to enable children and young people to design the research, carry it out and develop the analysis and findings (O'Kane, 2000). Such calls are as present in international research and work being done in the Global South as they are in research in the Global North (Abebe, 2009; Twum-Danso, 2009).

One of the many contributions that such research strategies and values provide is a counter balance to the contrasting priority found in institutionalised ethics procedures that emphasise children's vulnerability and need to be protected. Both procedures and ethical guidance regularly include children and young people within the sub-categories of research populations defined as vulnerable. The ESRC, who fund much of our work, is no exception (ESRC, 2015). Those who want to prioritise children and young people's capacity argue that such framings are problematic because they are used to justify working with adult others (often referred to as 'proxies') to explore children's lives and to acquiring consent from parents or other adult guardians rather than from children themselves (Davies, 2009; Morrow, 2005). Formal ethical procedures are still trapped in developmental understandings of children and childhood, which emphasise children's immaturity and incompetence. As Morrow and Richards argue:

> Arguments about ethics of social research with children can effectively be reduced to the question of the extent to which children are regarded as similar to or different from adults, and these discussions in turn can be reduced to two related descriptive perceptions that adults hold of children, that is, children as vulnerable and children as incompetent. These conceptualisations are reinforced by legal notions of childhood as a period of powerlessness and irresponsibility.
>
> (Morrow and Richards, 1996: 96)

In response, childhood researchers look to produce meaningful space where children and young people can make decisions about participation as a central value of their ethical practice. This does not necessarily mean that parental or adult consent is not still included (the children and young people themselves may want to include their parents or relevant adult carer in the consent process), but that adult consent is not seen as enough to ensure the children's best interests are protected. The priority is therefore shifted towards framing ethical practice as being about inclusion and participation, rather than protection from harm (Abebe, 2009). Such an approach does not deny issues of vulnerability, but instead re-locates vulnerability in social conditions and dynamics of power, which are best engaged with via participatory research methods, rather than traditional approaches to protection from research via minimising children's inclusion.

In some ways, one could argue that it is now the norm or even the orthodoxy that children should be involved in research about them. As McCarry (2012: 56) argues, 'social scientists no longer need to justify why CYP [children and young people] should be consulted but instead focus on how best to achieve this'. There are several positives that flow from this. Researchers have to give more robust accounts of why they would speak to adults rather than children when researching their lives. As in other areas of research, researchers also have to justify why it is worth taking up children and young people's time in order for their research to be undertaken. It is less easy (or should be) to say that children, or certain groups of children, are too hard to reach or work with. These moves are particularly important when thinking about disabled children and young people, where there has been a history of defining them as particularly vulnerable, hard to reach and limited in their ability to participate in research. The emphasis is now much more on developing the appropriate ways to both reach and work with them (Davis and Watson, 2001; Landsdown, 2001). As the call to involve children and young people in research has grown, concerns have been raised about the assumptions at times present within it. These queries are less about the specific techniques used, which are part of a wider, welcomed, move in social research to expand its methodological repertoire and value participatory possibilities, and more about how the ideas of childhood studies sit alongside the calls to value children and young people as experts in their own lives.

Childhood studies has at its centre the assertion that childhood is a heterogeneous social category, contingent in meaning and location. That beneath that social construction of 'childhood' live children and young people with many different lives, perspectives, understandings, informed by their particular cultural and material location. At the same time, the research practices that have emerged within childhood studies emphasise the capacity and agency children and young people have now – rather than in the future. That they can provide their own testimony about their social worlds. There seems a contradiction here between the conceptual claim that children are heterogeneous and socially located actors, and the political claim that they all have certain attributes as individual actors (James, 2007). Claims that children are experts in their own lives risk stripping children from the contexts that inform their understandings of their lives, individualising their accounts and their meanings (Gallacher and Gallagher, 2008; Gallagher, 2009). Gallacher and Gallagher (2008) have argued that the critique of developmental approaches that framed children as actors in a process of *becoming* subjects, has led to an over-fixation on claiming children are *beings* fully formed. While much of contemporary sociological research on adults emphasises the need to move away from thinking of subjects as individuals with certain capacities, at times, research on children and young people, through the wish to acknowledge their rights to participate in research and decisions about their lives, falls into naïve individualism. Such individualism carries the same problems that liberal rights holds for engaging fully with the inequalities adults face (this theme is returned to more fully in our final chapter). If research concentrates on what rights children as individuals have to participate, it may miss engaging with the social conditions that make their participation compromised. Leaving the assertion that they are being given research rights an empty one.

Other difficulties have been identified with the focus on children and young people as capable research subjects. Punch (2002b) highlights an inconsistency in the focus on children as fully-formed subjects, experts in their own lives, and the call made alongside that, that specific child-oriented techniques are required in order to empower them: 'If children are competent social actors, why are special 'child-friendly' methods needed to communicate with them?' (Punch, 2002b: 321). Recognising the heterogeneity of childhood and children also leaves in question that there are 'child-led', 'child-centred' or 'child-oriented' approaches (Hunleth, 2011). Do such techniques automatically work for all children, for all research and in all contexts? Is there a risk that calling things 'child-led' avoids engaging with thinking through how power is being engaged with, or how the varied social positionalities of children and young people will affect the research process? Hunleth (2011) argues that it is important that research claiming to be participatory in its approach to working with children, still question its practices and values. It should not assume that participatory techniques will always successfully tackle the complex power inequalities children face. When adult researchers seek approaches do they remain at the centre, aiming to empower children according to their measures of empowerment?

We would like to use creative methods as one area where these questions can be opened up. Are creative methods automatically more empowering for children? Why would we assume creative approaches are more emancipatory and interesting to all children and young people (Gibson *et al.*, 2013)? Hunleth (2011) has suggested that it is perhaps the adult researchers who like creative approaches, particularly when working on sensitive topics. She argues that creative methods enable adult researchers to avoid having to think about how to ask about such difficult issues within an interview context. Arguments that creative methods tap into children and young people's interest in storytelling and imagination, risk falling back into essentialist arguments that create false separations between adult and child modes of thinking and development. When we had planned to use creative methods – photography and artefact making – in the *Embodied Transitions* project, the aim had very much been to find techniques we thought young people would be more interested in and which would break out of the reliance on interviewing as our usual central research approach. Those who did participate in these different methods found them very interesting, and they did generate very rich and evocative material the interviews on their own would not have achieved. However, only a minority wished to participate in them. Seventeen participants took part in the interviews, eight became involved in the photography, six then followed that up with the photo-elicitation interview and finally three participated in the craft-making workshops. When participants opted to not participate in these multiple methods (which we fully supported them to do) the majority gave time as the reason they were happy to give (we acknowledge they may not have always wanted to give other reasons they may have had). Young people are busy, they spoke of exams and school work, of the other social and sport activities that filled their time. What they liked about the interview was it was a contained task, the more creative approaches took time they would have to take away from other things more important and meaningful to them. When we reflected on the preference for interviews we had a sense that for many of the participants they were comfortable with being asked for their thoughts; remembering, as we have observed, that disabled children and young people are not unfamiliar with having to explain their lives to adults. They were able to be reflective and critical about their own lives and this did not need to be mediated by other techniques. So while the photography, creative practice, and journals produced interesting material, interviews also did work with this group.

What our experiences on the *Embodied Transitions* project implies for us is that there is nothing essentially 'adult' (or child-unfriendly) about an interview, or child-centred about creative methods. Punch (2002b) argues that creative and innovative approaches can work with children, they can be fun and interesting, but this is because they can be that for any research participant. She therefore calls for them to be thought of as 'research-friendly' or 'person-friendly', rather than 'child-friendly', to avoid both homogenising all children as being the same and patronising them. The choice of research approach and technique should be drawn from consideration of the social contexts of the research, which informs the perspectives and understandings of those being researched, rather than assumed properties of the individuals involved in the study.

Conclusion

In Chapter 1 we made a case for thinking about children as relational actors, embedded in a range of social networks through which dynamics of power, regulation and situated agency emerge. This understanding means that we are wary of treating research with children as a distinct process in seeking out children and young people's authentic voice and expertise. Instead, we would argue that the voices and expertise children and young people enact in their lives or in research practice are produced and are emergent within the networks they are part of, including the research itself as an interactional network. Their capacity and expertise is produced through their interactions with others. One aspect this can effect – as an example – is the role of others, formally and informally, in consent processes. While we always seek consent from children and young people themselves (sometimes, although not always, alongside consent from a parent or adult guardian), we are conscious of how their decision can be influenced by others. It is not enough to ask for their consent, it is important to look broadly at the setting in which they are making 'their' decision, Parents may want their children to participate and try to persuade them to agree, or may encourage their child's own sense of self and aim for a space for the decision to be theirs. Disabled children and young people's experiences of health and social care may make them overly familiar with giving consent in such a way that they do not think through what is being asked of them (just another adult asking them stuff), or it may make them particularly able to scrutinise the researcher and research, asking pertinent questions of what is being asked of them.

We can understand why, politically, much has been made of children and young people's abilities; this has been needed as a counterbalance to presumptions that they are inherently incapable, incompetent. However, the cost has been the creation of an equally fictional abstract character held apart from the social worlds that is shaping them. To us, it is important that research engage with the relational networks children and young people are participants in – including the worlds of adults. The worlds of children are not completely separate domains; seeing them as participants in shaping their worlds does not mean adults are not present. Again, this seems counter to the recognition that children are surveyed, controlled and regulated through the spaces they move through and institutions they are contained within. This is no more so than for disabled children and young people who will often spend more time with adults than other children and young people. This is both because their interactions with actors such as health and social care professionals will be more frequent and also because their opportunities to be freely in public and social spaces away from adults will be less common. None of this means that ideas about working appropriately with children and young people are not valuable, or that a focus on gaining their permission to be where they are is not more ethical. Rather it is to question this as particular to children and young people. These are important norms for working with any group of research participants. The focus should be in understanding the relationships and interactions that inform the social issues and actors being examined, and in developing ways to engage with those relationships and interactions. This includes the adults who are, due to the worlds we live in, part of those relationships and interactions. For this reason we would see our work as – at least aiming towards – the ethnographic practices others advocate for their ability to study 'embodied relations and practices' (Woodyer, 2008: 352). This enables both relationality to be engaged with in the interactions observed, and also the non-verbal presence of young children to be acknowledged as significant to the networks they are part of.

References

Abebe, T. (2009) Multiple methods, complex dilemmas: negotiating socio-ethical spaces in participatory research with disadvantaged children. *Children's Geographies*, 7(4): 451–465.

Alderson, P. (2001) Research by children. *International Journal of Social Research Methodology*, 4(2): 139–153.

Bagnoli, A. (2011) Making sense of mixed method narratives: young people's identities, life-plans and orientations. In S. Heath and C. Walker (eds), *Innovations in Youth Research*. pp. 77–100. Basingstoke: Palgrave Macmillan.

Christensen, P. (2004) Children's participation in ethnographic research: issues of power and representation. *Children & Society*, 18(2): 165–176.

Christensen, P. and James, A. (eds) (2000) *Research with Children: Perspectives and Practices*. London and New York, NY: Falmer Press.

Clavering, E.K. and McLaughlin, J. (2010) Children's participation in health research: from objects to agents? *Child: Care, Health and Development*, 36(5): 603–611.

Darbyshire, P., MacDougall, C. and Schiller, W. (2005) Multiple methods in qualitative research with children: more insight or just more? *Qualitative Research*, 5(4): 417–436.

Davies, H. (2009) Reflexivity in research practice: informed consent with children at school and at home. *Sociological Research Online*, 13(4): www.socresonline.org.uk/13/4/5.html

Davis, J.M. and Watson, N. (2001) Where are the children's experiences? Analysing social and cultural exclusion in 'special' and 'mainstream' schools. *Disability & Society*, 16(5): 671–687.

ESRC (2015) *ESRC Framework for Research Ethics* www.esrc.ac.uk/files/funding/guidance-for-applicants/esrc-framework-for-research-ethics-2015/

Franklin, A. and Sloper, P. (2006) *Participation of Disabled Children and Young People in Decision-Making Relating to Social Care*. York: Social Policy Research Unit.

Gallacher, L.-A. and Gallagher, M. (2008) Methodological immaturity in childhood research? Thinking through 'participatory methods'. *Childhood*, 15(4): 499–516.

Gallagher, M. (2009) Rethinking participatory methods in children's geographies. In L. van Blerk and M. Kesby (eds), *Doing Children's Geographies: Methodological Issues in Research with Young People*. pp. 84–97. London: Routledge.

Gibson, B.E., Bhavnita, M., Smith, B., Yoshida, K.K., Abbott, D. and Lindsay, S. (2013) The integrated use of audio diaries, photography, and interviews with research with disabled young men. *International Journal of Qualitative Methods*, 12: 383–402.

Hart, R. (1992) *Children's Participation: From Tokenism to Citizenship.* UNICEF: www. unicef-irc.org/publications/pdf/childrens_participation.pdf

Hunleth, J. (2011) Beyond on or with: questioning power dynamics and knowledge production in 'child-oriented' research methodology. *Childhood*, 18(1): 81–93.

James, A. (2007) Giving voice to children's voices: practices and problems, pitfalls and potentials. *American Anthropologist*, 109(2): 261–272.

Kellett, M. (2005) *Children as Active Researchers: A New Research Paradigm for the 21st Century?* Swindon: ESRC.

Kellett, M. (2010) *Rethinking Children and Research.* London: Continuum.

Kullman, K. (2012) Experiments with moving children and digital cameras. *Children's Geographies*, 10(1): 1–16.

Landsdown, G. (2001) *It is Our World Too! A Report on the Lives of Disabled Children.* Disability Awareness in Action: www.daa.org.uk/uploads/pdf/It%20is%20Our%20 World%20Too!.pdf

Mason, J. and Hood, S. (2010) Exploring issues of children as actors in social research. *Children and Youth Services Review*, 33: 490–495.

McCarry, M. (2012) Who benefits? A critical reflection of children and young people's participation in sensitive research. *International Journal of Social Research Methodology*, 15(1): 55–68.

McLaughlin, J., Goodley, D., Clavering, E.K. and Fisher, P. (2008) *Families Raising Disabled Children: Enabling Care and Social Justice.* Basingstoke: Palgrave Macmillan.

Melton, G.B., Ben-Arieh, A., Cashmore, J., Goodman, G.␣. and Worley, N.K. (eds) (2013) *The Sage Handbook of Child Research.* London: Sage.

Morrow, V. (2001) Using qualitative methods to elicit young people's perspectives on their environments: some ideas for community health initiatives. *Health Education Research*, 16(3): 255–268.

Morrow, V. (2005) Ethical issues in collaborative research with children. In A. Farrell (ed.), *Ethical Research with Children.* pp. 150–165. Maidenhead: Open University Press.

Morrow, V. and Richards, M. (1996) The ethics of social research with children: an overview. *Children & Society*, 10: 90–105.

Nabors, L.A. (2013) *Research Methods for Children.* New York, NY: Nova Science Publishers.

O'Kane, C. (2000) The development of participatory techniques: facilitating children's views about decisions which affect them. In P. Christensen and A. James (eds), *Research with Children: Perspectives and Practices.* pp. 125–156. London: Routledge.

Punch, S. (2002a) Interviewing strategies with young people: the 'secret box', stimulus material and task-based activities. *Children & Society*, 16: 45–56.

Punch, S. (2002b) Research with children: the same or different from research with adults? *Childhood*, 9(3): 321–341.

Save the Children (2000) *Young People as Researchers.* London: Save the Children.

Save the Children (2004) *So You Want to Involve Children in Research? A Toolkit Supporting Children's Meaningful and Ethical Participation in Research Relating to Violence against Children.* Stockholm, Sweden: Save the Children.

Shaw, C., Brady, L.-M. and Davey, C. (2011) *Guidelines for Research with Children and Young People.* London: National Children's Bureau.

Sutherland, H. and Young, A. (2014) Research with deaf children and not on them: a study of method and process. *Children & Society*, 28(5): 366–379.

Todd, L. (2012) Critical dialogue, critical methodology: bridging the research gap to young people's participation in evaluating children's services. *Children's Geographies*, 10(2): 187–200.

Twum-Danso, A. (2009) Situating participatory methodologies in context: the impact of culture on adult-child interactions in research and other projects. *Children's Geographies*, 7(4): 379–389.

Valentine, G. (1999) Being seen and heard? The ethical complexities of working with young people at home and at school. *Ethics, Place and Environment*, 2: 141–155.

Warming, H. (2011) Getting under their skins? Accessing young children's perspectives through ethnographic fieldwork. *Childhood*, 18(1): 39–53.

Woodyer, T. (2008) The body as research tool: embodied practice and children's geographies. *Children's Geographies*, 6(4): 349–362.

Part II
Monitoring institutions

3   Institutional norms and transitions

Understanding disabled childhoods requires making sense of how key institutions of childhood generate concepts and practices about normal ways of being, acting and thinking. Central here is education where the policies and practices of schooling guide learning in line with normative standards of development and achievement. It also refers to an ideal: the desire for children to have access to opportunities for socially beneficial learning organised in accordance to standards of the normal, and to share in those opportunities at the same time, in the same place, and in the same way. Outside of childhood, the mainstream refers to cultural institutions of adulthood that structure imaginaries around children's futures. People are expected to aspire to economic and social independence, employment and a family life (heterosexual coupledom, monogamy and reproduction). Practices that stand outside of the normal, including sexual and intimate practices that fail to conform to normative standards (Warner, 1999), and forms of social participation that are not valued in the same way as paid employment (such as care), are frequently excluded. Visions of normality in childhood and the marking out of a normal adult life, by disabled children and young people and by their families, is the central focus of this chapter.

As discussed in Chapter 1, our interest in normality is based on a concern with the consequences of falling away from what is considered to be a normal human existence. Understandings of normality matter because differing from social expectations of what constitutes the normal can have significant consequences for someone's recognition as a valued and legitimate social actor (Honneth, 1996; Kittay, 2006). We follow Foucault's (1990, 1991) argument that modernity has been marked by the move away from the maintenance of social order through overt state control to processes of regulation, which establish the normal, including targeting the troublesome for rehabilitation and requiring the individual to self-regulate both body and mind. State mechanisms inform the delineation of normality, but the dynamic of governmentality occurs equally at the level of self-monitoring and disciplining people's own practice.

Disability is a core category in establishing the normality of persons and practices – it is not so much normality that establishes disability; but rather through identifying what is considered the strange, the ill-fitting, and the unacceptable, the normal and the normativity of that normal is established. Our approach to normality is to understand it as constructed through a number of processes, which draw together the overlapping influence of institutions, cultural and material practices and discursive categorisations that help produce boundaries between ways of being, looking and acting that are positioned as normal or abnormal. Medicine's role in these processes is the focus of the next chapter, here we will focus on education and the transitions to the institutions of adulthood and their role in securing categories of difference which bring with them judgement and marginalisation.

It is helpful to keep in mind locations outside the Global North as including within them different narratives and practices to those that inform accounts of work done here (Clark *et al.*, 2010; Grant and Furstenberg, 2007). For example, as will be discussed later in this chapter, a key norm in transitions from adolescence to adulthood in most Global North contexts is the shift from living with family (assumed to be parents and siblings) to living on one's own, before then establishing one's own nuclear family. Looking outside the Global North this version of transition is not necessarily central to young people's lives, although some argue it is becoming so under the influence of globalisation. In Asian contexts patterns of extended family living can change (in gendered ways) as someone moves into adulthood, but living with particular sets of changing extended family relations throughout that transition and into adulthood can be part of the norm. Rao (2001), drawing from research undertaken in India, argues that such patterns of extended family living can be influential in the integration of disabled members into family life as normal and not particularly noteworthy. In such contexts she also argues that the need to categorise variations in mind-body capabilities into categories of disability appear less important: the more expansive the boundaries of normality, the less the need to provide categories of difference. Therefore, in exploring the institutional production of categories of normality in this chapter, we acknowledge that these are norms very much situated in the Global North.

The first part explores the presence of material and cultural norms within schooling (mainstream and special) and how they operate to mark out disabled children and young people as both different and troublesome. The second part considers how both parents and disabled children and young people imagine their adult futures and the insight that generates of what are thought of as the normal futures to aspire to within the institutions of adulthood.

Schooling normality

For all young people schools are key institutions in which normality is learnt. Education can be thought of as a site of governmentality where 'all young children are perceived to need to learn the norms that govern society' (Holt *et al.*, 2012: 2192). One objective of educational inclusion is to create a greater variety of person, styles of learning, and modes of interaction within mainstream educational spaces. However, the presence of governmentality practices may instead mean that mainstream education settings provide both opportunities for children and young people with mind-body differences (Holt's (2004a) mind-body formulation, which we highlighted in The Introduction, is particularly useful to work with in this chapter) to be categorised as disabled and to be worked on to improve their fit with established categories of normality. Cross cultural analyses of educational curriculum have suggested that the Global North's focus on the provision of linguistic and logical skills, encourages the perception that those who struggle with these specific skills are disabled in ways that would not occur in different curriculum contexts (Gardner, 1993; Harry and Kalyanpur, 1994). The category of disability is produced in a mode of education that sets the boundaries of what normal learning and functioning is (Madriaga *et al.*, 2011).

Visible educational priorities also sit alongside unwritten goals of educational practice, which can also prioritise normality in problematic ways. For example, the concept of the 'hidden curriculum' is used by critical education researchers to suggest that what lies behind formal goals of education such as literacy and numeracy are attempts to produce the right kinds of future citizens. Ashby (2010: 350) argues that this hidden goal influences an approach to the education of disabled children that prioritises minimising 'the effects of the disability, to do things more the way able-bodied people do them; in fact to make the person more normal'. Davis and Watson (2001) have highlighted the ways in which, through reward and punishment, disabled young people are taught to conform to certain ways of thinking and doing that are valorised in school contexts – for example being able to sit quietly in rows, while responding to specific requests by teachers (Nadesan, 2005). Those who then struggle to comply with such practices are more likely to be defined as unruly, difficult and abnormal.

Ethnographic research is invaluable in capturing such practices and the work of Holt and her colleagues in both primary and secondary mainstream and special educational contexts has produced a detailed picture of the micropolitics of this complex social space for children with mind-body differences. Most countries in the Global North have made some level of transition from primarily or solely educating disabled children separately in 'special schools', towards policies of integration and inclusion within mainstream educational environments (Vlachou, 1997). However, Holt's UK research highlights how previous practices of segregation have found their way into mainstream educational spaces as '[d]iscourses of (dis)ability ... are reproduced through everyday practices within classroom spaces' (Holt, 2004a: 220), producing new forms of 'micro exclusions within school spaces' (Holt *et al.*, 2012: 2196). Micro-exclusions occur through a number of practices. First, the tradition of keeping disabled children separate in different institutions continues in mainstream spaces when they are located away from other children in the class room, in playgrounds, and in special break out spaces. Second, the provision of support for disabled children can become a symbol of their difference through how they are supplied with different kinds of materials, the visible presence of learning support teachers and through how they come in and out of the class room in order to have 'special attention' such as physiotherapy or speech and language therapy. Third, children with mind-body differences in mainstream educational spaces can find themselves judged as different and other through the dominance of normal models of childhood development (Holt, 2004b). The 'proper purpose' of mainstream education – of helping the 'normal' development of children in reaching goals of learning and maturity – positions the child with mind-body differences as outside the norm and a problem to the normal goals of the school (Holloway and Valentine, 2000). Finally, children themselves pick up institutional patterns of othering through segregation by replicating, and at times extending, such segregations in their own understandings of themselves and each other in social interactions in the classroom and outside it.

One of the several problematic outcomes of such (dis)abling practices is the way that normative expectations of child behaviour help to facilitate the production of 'self-regulating subjects' (Holt, 2004a: 227) who subsequently do the work of modifying behaviour to approximate such norms. This work is often targeted towards those with differences categorised as within Autistic Spectrum Disorder, for example, '[t]eaching the young people on the AS [Autistic Spectrum] to learn to cooperate, to correct their perceived deficiencies (rather than focusing on their talents and abilities' (Holt *et al.*, 2012: 2199). This can lead such children to work towards the norms they are said to fail. Naraian and Natarajan (2013) have undertaken similar research in India as schools have in recent years made steps towards integration. They found disabled children seeking to act like those around them in order to be both accepted and seen as normal. However, one problem they faced in this quest is that the school settings themselves were so unaccommodating to their needs that it was impossible for them to be read as normal – not because of anything to do with them, but because their 'inclusive environment' marked them as different and other.

The exclusionary practices of either children or adults do not necessarily emerge from conscious attempts to exclude and marginalise those who are different. They develop from wider pressures on schools (not least from the pressure on schools to excel academically), from the incorporation of dominant norms from wider society, from the long history of the segregation of those identified as different into 'other' spaces, and from the power of standards of normality in shaping the politics of everyday interaction and recognition across society. The emergence of exclusionary practices through such routes is hard to challenge, but also holds open the possibility of change as people find new ways of engaging with each other and responding to difference within the heterogeneous spaces of the school environment (Olin and Jansson, 2009):

> Although individuals cannot, perhaps, fully escape the terms of reference within which they become subjects, subjectivities can be interpreted in a variety of ways within these terms of reference. 'Acceptable' subjectivities establish the *limits* to how identities can be performed without transgression, rather than *determining* practice. Consequently, teachers and students perform ability and disability slightly differently in different classroom micro-spaces.
>
> (original emphasis, Holt, 2004a: 226)

Norms are made real in their practice; while mainstream schools may seek to hold on to their pre-existing norms, the presence of others who engage with those practices in different ways cannot help but open up at least the possibility of their transformation. In the gaps between exclusionary practice, opportunities where both child and adult–child relationships are 'punctuated by aspects of connection and difference' become possible. While childhood cultures can be exclusionary and hierarchical, they also can be 'supportive and nurturing' (Holt, 2004a: 230). In such moments of connection an imaginary is glimpsed which could 'deconstruct binary divisions between disability and non-disability' (Holt, 2004a: 234). Such 'momentary transformations' have the 'immanent political potential to expand the norms by which society is governed within specific school spaces' (Holt *et al.*, 2012: 2193) and hold open the possibility that norms could be expanded to recognise broader possibilities of 'which lives are liveable' (Holt *et al.*, 2012: 2202).

Fitting into the mainstream

The distinction between subjects of inclusion and subjects of exclusion has long structured the experience of schooling in the Global North, and judgements made against children 'regarded as exceptional' (Winzer, 1993: 3) have been the basis on which disabled children have been segregated within the institutional spaces of education. In a context of integration, the relation of the 'exceptional' to the normal becomes one of accommodation. Disabled children get 'integrated' by schools looking to accommodate them in structures intended for non-disabled children. This is shaped by a range of modalities, including how schools are designed, how teachers are trained, and how children are expected to behave and learn. The privileging of particular bodies, behaviours and learning styles orient the gaze towards those children who less successfully embody the norm, and informs understandings of disabled children as requiring special forms of monitoring control.

In our own research we have seen a variety of school based practices that have penalised disabled children and young people for their apparent inability to enact normality. The school response often has been to seek to mould the children to the pre-existing standards they appear to struggle to achieve and which the educational system defines as important. We will give three examples here, from a broader set of practices that serve to differentiate disabled children and young people in mainstream schooling contexts. First, from nurseries onwards parents seeking mainstream education for their children have struggled to find spaces that would let their children be present in ways different to usual disciplining practice:

> I was told by one of the other mothers that during coffee break 'we like the children to sit quietly at the table over there'. Then during singsong time, all the kids were expected to sit cross-legged on the floor. Totally not Duncan's place!
>
> (Interview Two, Duncan's Mum, *Enabling Care* project)

The sense of the disabled mind-body as disordered also emerges around concerns with risk. In the *Enabling Care* project we worked with Frank's family (Frank had a permanent tracheotomy in his throat) while they sought to find an appropriate nursery environment for him. At the first nursery we observed teachers so scared of the responsibility of caring for both the equipment and Frank, that they presented him as a constant threat to them and himself:

> Just about the first thing the support worker spoke about relating to Frank was her anxiety around the implications for her around his tracheotomy – she was very aware that she had to be watching him constantly to ensure there was no blockage. When she was speaking to me about this she was fidgeting quite a bit and it made me very conscious of how unsettled she appeared to be. She also spoke about this later in the day when we were outside with Frank who was playing with the sand tray something that appeared to put her yet more on edge. Although Frank had a cotton cover to protect the trachy valve from getting blocked, she spoke of a high risk of sand granules getting through the gauze and blocking his airways. The possibility of this happening, and her own concerns around her responsibility to Frank and worries about the need to be constantly vigil meant that she hovered near to him and checked the way other children played around him with heavy emphasis on making sure no one got carried away with their playing so sand was not chucked around.
>
> (Observation notes of Frank at Nursery, *Enabling Care* project)

The contemporary emphasis given to managing and avoiding risk in schools creates a context which defines Frank as troublesome.

A second area where the disabled mind-body is troubling to normal schooling is around how schools seek to accommodate disabled children within existing physical education (PE) provision. In the *Embodied Transitions* project, a number of the young people we interviewed who attended mainstream schools told us about their experiences of PE and how they found PE to be a key site where their difference from other pupils were reinforced. They spoke of how they were placed in non-active roles such as being a referee or keeping scores, or alternatively playing in a way that was vastly different to how other children played. As a result of these efforts at accommodation, the young people's sense of themselves was that they were out-of-place, or not wholly part of what was going on around them:

> ...in PE you're always, like the teacher had last year, they always used to ask me the questions 'cos obviously I couldn't take part and he wanted to make sure I was listening, so he used to say, 'So how does so and so stand like this?' and I'd be half asleep I had no idea, and I'm not interested in sport but, so that was a bit annoying 'cos I used to get asked, 'You need to be paying attention', oh right fine, even watch, and it's always refereeing they're always saying 'Why don't you referee a game? Why don't you count

the score?' and I'm like I've done that twenty million times, it's always the same things and I'm just not interested in sport at all.

(Interview One, Sean, *Embodied Transitions* project)

A final aspect we want to highlight of how schools can fail to work with the disabled mind-body generating 'micro-exclusion' lies within the physical inaccessibility of 'inclusive' schools. Contemporary public spaces, including most mainstream schools, continue to be designed in ways that assume the 'normality of the non-disabled body' (Imrie, 2013: 3448). The inclusion of disabled people is often, as Imrie notes, an 'afterthought', and integration typically gets achieved through adaptation after a space is built. In the childhood SPARCLE interviews in the *Embodied Transitions* project, Kate talked of the difficulties she had both moving around her school and being with her friends due to the lack of space for the frame she used to help her walk:

INTERVIEWER: Is there anywhere else at school that the frame, gets in the way of you going there?

KATE: Often, 'cos in our classroom, we have like, say this is one table [miming tables spaced out] and then we have a gap and then we have another table and then we have a gap and then we have another table, well often I can't get through there with my frame. Often that's where all my friends sit and stuff so...

INTERVIEWER: Yeah, and have you told them that you can't get there?

KATE: Yeah, I've told them that and also in the dining hall, there's just a very small gap of seats in the dining hall so I often can't get to sit with my friends. 'cos very often I have to sit on the end which is a place I can get on.

(SPARCLE Childhood Interview, Kate, *Embodied Transitions* project)

One of the interesting things about Kate's account is that she defines the problem as the frame, rather than either the inaccessibility of the school environment or the unresponsiveness of her friends – both of which if configured differently would enable her to be the subject of inclusion. Defining the problem as being her frame and by connection, her, means that her own body is understood as the source of her marginalisation in the social space of school:

KATE: It's good to be different but I hate having [whispers] my disability

INTERVIEWER: What is it that you hate about it, do you think?

KATE: I've got to take this big frame thing around with me and in the playground there's a set of steps and my friends always go round the back onto the set of steps and because I have to trail this thing around with me I can't get down the steps so I can't play with my friends a lot of the time because [whispers] they are on the steps.

(SPARCLE Childhood Interview, Kate, *Embodied Transitions* project)

This was a common framing; the problems were often understood as within their minds-bodies and their lack of fit with the environment. It was also reinforced in the relation of the disabled children to the better accommodated and less restricted able-bodied children around them:

> SARA: That I can't really do things that other people, that other people could do like I'd quite like to be doing skateboarding and roller skating and ballet
>
> …
>
> INTERVIEWER: What would you like to happen when you're older?
>
> SARA: I'd quite like to walk.
>
> (SPARCLE Childhood Interview, Sara, *Embodied Transitions* project)

In response to being presented as the carriers of difference, the most common response by research participants was to seek to minimise symbols of difference – such as not using the big frame if possible – as a strategy of normalisation that aimed to place disability into the background. In Chapter 5 we will talk about this in detail in terms of how disabled children and young people and their families sought to manage their embodied difference and the technologies that supported their bodies. What we can highlight here is the way it led to discomfort with help and support as symbols of difference and abnormality:

> Dad had to take us on that [school trip to local holiday resort] and it was a lovely day but I wasn't looking forward to it at all because literally half the school were going, and me dad would have to push me round and I suppose I still feel the same, it was a nice day at the end of it but I was determined not to go at first and then I managed to go, but I was determined not to 'cos it's just felt a bit out of the fashion, I mean all the other parents weren't there 'cos me dad, 'cos they all got buses, whereas my dad drove me there which was very kind of him.
>
> (Interview One, Sean, *Embodied Transitions* project)

The wish to be seen as normal contributed to a dislike of markers of support – the frame, the father taking you on a school trip. It also encouraged any actions which appeared to be located in someone's wish to 'help out' the disabled child to be seen as patronising and othering:

> …like taking a penalty, this has happened to me quite a lot. People know obviously you couldn't be able to hit the ball like a hundred mile an hour but you take the shot and it's an easy save and people like dive over the ball and let it go in it's like it's a bit of cringing sort of thing, just save the ball, man. Stop taking the mick. Whenever I do it, because they think it's gonna get like help me more I'd rather them just save the ball and say yeah it wasn't a very good penalty or it wasn't a very good shot at saving the ball it's an easy save like most people dive over the ball or slip over and it's just, c'mon you're taking the mick.
>
> (Interview One, Mark, *Embodied Transitions* project)

Several were unhappy with the presence of a learning support worker, including Kate who in her first interview with us at 15 explained she had requested the removal of her worker because she wanted to learn to be independent like other pupils and disliked how the worker positioned her as different. Requiring additional help is itself not a problem; this is what we would like to think friends and family do for us. However, the issue here is how such forms of help are (a) a product of an inaccessible environment and (b) direct the gaze of difference because they differ from the normal ways things are done. Mainstream schools can, therefore, in their approach to inclusion, mark disabled children as different through the ways in which they respond to varied needs and produce an environment that requires additional help to navigate.

One clear outcome of such negative experiences or perceptions of mainstream space is that disabled children themselves can favour special education. In our research special schools were seen as safe because they could avoid 'people there [mainstream school] who don't really like people like me' (Interview One, Andrew, *Embodied Transitions* project). In special education – including in some cases in the safety of special units in mainstream schools – some participants felt comfortable as they were schooled with others who had, as Lauren said, 'different stuff that's the matter with them' (One-Off Interview, Lauren, *Embodied Transitions* project). Special education was identified as a place where they did not need to pretend to be normal by hiding their disability:

> If I went to say a mainstream, my main concern would be me getting bullied. Because of my disability that would be my main concern, 'cos I have been called names in the past by people. And I would be concerned they might push me or pick on me because of my disability…. Yeah I've been called lovely names, and because, I've been called some lovely names in the past and if they called me names or picked on me I would get really down, and I know that. 'Cos to me when I'm out places I tend to hide my disability, try to hide it.
>
> (Interview One, Hannah, *Embodied Transitions* project)

Special schools were also favoured because of the increased level of support they would receive there (support which again would not define them as different as high levels of support were the norm):

> In a normal school you wouldn't get, see I get help with writing, reading and maths, my English, science. If I was in a normal school say a class of thirty kids I wouldn't get that. 'Cos it's thirty kids with one teacher and one support teacher, where here there's more than one support teacher and, and they can sit down with you, help you if you need it, read to you.
>
> (Interview One, Ryan, *Embodied Transitions* project)

However, special schools do not always integrate children with different disabilities well either. Schools for disabled children construct their own cultures of normality, as well as hierarchies of impairment, marking out some as belonging and others as unwelcome. Hannah, for instance, described her feelings when her school was turned into what she described as a school for autistic children and not physically disabled children like her. This change jeopardised the inclusive environment she had once experienced:

> there was quite a lot of changes going on in our school, then it used to be for physically disabled kids like me, but now it's for autism and we shouldn't be mixed, 'cos we got different needs and that wasn't great, having physically disabled kids like me mixed with autism, it's completely different … it wasn't suitable for me anymore, like [pause] and the kids some kids were pretty violent too … I did get whacked a couple of times off kids, the kids with autism, because they lash out.
>
> (Interview One, Hannah, *Embodied Transitions* project)

While from the young people's perspective the valuing of special schooling is understandable there is reason to problematize their choice, both for what it means for them and for future disabled young people. The favouring of special education is a logical result of practices within mainstream settings that appear unable, or unwilling to approach making an environment inclusive of differences. When support is provided in a way that demarcates some as in need and others as not, this is a product of an environment that is hostile to difference and unwilling to move away from a prescriptive curriculum that measures success within narrow parameters. The difficulty for the child or young person, or for the parent/carer, is that the current structuring of mainstream schooling leaves them with very imperfect choices, which may help maintain or even encourage the continued presence of segregation in special schools and poor levels of inclusion in mainstream. The problem is not so much with the possibility that different children require different kinds of educational environments and interactions, but with how those differences are marginalised in mainstream environments because standards of normality hold precedence.

Holt and colleagues (2013) argue that there can be practices within mainstream school that do fracture the hegemonic power of exclusionary norms. Across our research projects we have seen practices that approach differences in innovative and imaginary ways, which provide templates for how the norms of how we do things and why can be expanded to include greater variety. It is possible for school spaces, teaching, and curricula to be made expansive of diversity. Sometimes they required additional resources, most often they involved imagination, creativity and, most importantly, flexibility in how the school operated. Sean in the *Embodied Transitions* project at the time of his second interview was preparing for surgery that would interrupt his preparations for key school exams and his ability to take the exams at their usual times. Rather than force him to repeat the year, the school was altering the examination process to enable greater use of course work and alternative times for exams so he could carry on. Rachel spoke in her second *Embodied Transitions* interview of a key

PE teacher who had always found ways for her to be included in lessons (in the process encouraging her interest in sport which continued post schooling):

INTERVIEWER: So is it important that you were integrated into that…?
RACHEL: Yeah and even though I did it slightly different I was still involved in the activities and that so I was always involved and you know I was never left out or anything like that.

(Interview Two, Rachel, *Embodied Transitions* project)

Earlier we mentioned the problems Frank experienced in nursery when teachers and assistants positioned him as different because of his tracheotomy and his different mode of communication. The marginalisation Frank experienced led his mother to transfer him to another nursery where his treatment was transformed, enabling him to become a full participant in that space. Training was put in place so they were fully confident in how to look after his trachy and tube. In addition, the speech and language therapist who was teaching him Makaton showed the other children how to use some of the signs too, so nursery communication as a norm included periods of using Makaton. Things changed again when Frank started primary school; a framework of celebrating difference and inclusion created a space where Frank's differences were supported by both staff and pupils, enabling him to be a full participant in the school space:

The school and particularly the learning support woman is fantastic, very confident, she instils confidence, she's even said if Frank's back on oxygen she has no problem with him going into school on his oxygen. And the school have been great, they're very supportive, it's a school which embraces difference as just part of life and they do a lot of things.

(Interview Three, Frank's Mum, *Enabling Care* project)

Teachers and catering staff had been trained up on how to look after his tracheotomy and the learning support worker provided for Frank was integrated into the classroom in a way that meant it was not immediately obvious that she was 'Frank's':

The learning support teacher specifically for Frank and for nobody else. But she does it in a way where she's not, she helps out in the class, so she's like a classroom assistant but she has her eye on Frank all the time and Frank's development and integration and everything, so he doesn't feel as if, [pause] to everybody she's just another member, is the second teacher in the class. She's not Frank's, nobody knows.

(Interview Three, Frank's Mum, *Enabling Care* project)

The creativity of the space made it possible to shift from Frank having to be the one accommodating to normal practice; instead practice was accommodated to him in a way that no longer identified his presence as problematic.

Much work remains to be done to ensure education provides an arena where disabled children and young people can be full participants. Here we concentrated on how issues around the ways in which disabled bodies were made to be out of place via the ways schools can be designed and organised and the emphasis given to things such as conformativity and physical education. However, as other researchers such as Holt have identified, there can also be ways in which schools respond that can challenge such exclusionary practices. Some of this is about everyday practices that seek to find new ways of doing things; it is also about a shift in culture which works to create institutional environments that see difference as within the normal and something to be celebrated and encouraged rather than accommodated to. One important role of education is to prepare children for the transition to adulthood, embedded in that preparation are norms about what that future adulthood will involve. Next we look at some of those expectations about the future and what is involved in a successful transition, from the perspective of parents and carers and disabled children and young people.

Transitions and imagined futures

Transition is a key concept in work on disability and young people and youth studies; in particular the transition from adolescence to adulthood. Bringing both areas of work together can aid greater appreciation of how key norms are embedded in transitions. In particular it can enable us to capture how key institutions of adulthood such as work and family are important in policing the norms of appropriate and valued transition. In work on disability a predominant theme (changing somewhat with the influence of critical disability studies) has been the transition from child services (in health and social care) to adult services and the lack of appropriate transition planning and support that occurs. A theme that is also shared with work looking at other children and young people involved in state supported care who are faced with 'sudden adulthood' (Rogers, 2011). Those researching disability have highlighted how disability 'troubles' pathways to adulthood. Moola and Norman (2011) provide a useful summary of such accounts that details some of the barriers disabled young people face, such as parental over protection, institutional failures to support transitions, stigma and prejudice. However, Moola and Norman argue that this research has failed to interrogate the concept of *the transition to adulthood*, assuming an established normal pathway that people would move through if disability was not there. Such an understanding then implies that the solution is to help disabled young people to move on to that correct pathway, through which happiness and success will be found. Such work makes the mistake of assuming that 'the movement from adolescence to adulthood is a one-time intractable event' (Moola and Norman, 2011: 842), which can be obtained for disabled people with just the right kind of institutional response. In doing so the relational dynamics of transition as a complex form of identity making and remaking are ignored (Gillies, 2000) and its underlying disciplinary norms left un-critiqued.

Therefore, disability makes a difference not just in providing a different set of organisational and institutional contexts and social barriers (which is true), but also a different relationship to understandings of transitions. For example, one version of the norm of successful transition is to become a productive adult citizen, through both contributing to the workplace and raising a family. If this norm is not questioned for disabled young people, then the problem with transition is ensuring that no barriers exist to them obtaining that social position. What is left unquestioned is whether this is the only form of successful transition through which someone can become an adult and be recognised as such. In addition, this way of framing transition also seeks validation in the future. A certainty is presented that that future will be obtained. But the impairments and illnesses some young people live with may mean that their future may not be clear or lived within that presumed time frame. Holding the importance of being young is the transition you make during it, avoids recognising the present as being of value in itself.

Youth studies has a broader focus, but one which has significantly failed to take an interest in disability as a social location, discursive construct and troubling embodied identity that matters to transition dynamics. It is a great loss that youth studies has shown little interest in incorporating disability into their work on transitions (Coles, 2000). This is not just because disability provides a different setting for youth transition, more importantly a consideration of disability supports the work going on in youth studies to problematize understandings of transition in complex and changing times (Rogers, 2011): 'the heterogeneity of childhoods and adulthoods can serve to critique and destabilise dominant representations of childhood as a ubiquitous route from dependent infanthood to independent adulthood' (Holt, 2004b).

Much of the current work in youth studies is about providing an explanation for why transitions to adulthood are becoming more fractured, fluid and uncertain (Bradley and Devadason, 2008; Dwyer and Wyn, 2001; Holdsworth and Morgan, 2005; Jones *et al.*, 2006). Indeed MacDonald (2011) argues that because of young people's location between different social and institutional worlds, studying their transitions is a valuable way of monitoring societal change within employment, family living and other areas of social life. One stream of this work is to analyse trends in socio-economic patterns of young people's lives in order to capture changes in areas such as education (staying in further and higher education is increasingly a norm for a broader range of young people), employment (it now takes longer to find stable employment), and living arrangements (people now leave the family home later and return more often and live for longer in patterns of shared living and transient co-habitation before 'settling down'). Arnett (2004) has referred to the more staggered, unstable and varied transitions as representing an elongation of adolescence into a period of 'emerging adulthoods' through which the responsibilities of 'full adulthood' are legitimately delayed in contexts such as higher education, travelling and exploring different forms of employment and consumption.

Another stream in youth studies takes as its focus the cultural shifts occurring in young people's lives (Furlong *et al.*, 2011). This work argues that the cultural lives of young people are of interest and value in and of themselves, and that transitions across childhood, adolescence and adulthood have always been (without denying that change is occurring in the Global North) more varied and complex than the institutional processes of transition from school to work, or family living to living on one's own would suggest (Worth, 2009). Such work seeks to capture the significance of people's relational lives and agency in responding to the shifts in socio-economic institutions they are experiencing (Wierenga, 2011).

Drawing cultural dynamics into analyses of the changing socio-economic contexts of transitions in contemporary social worlds enables us to think about adulthood as a category achieved by acquiring, through involvement in various institutions, the symbols, practices, resources, and outlook that others recognise as being its markers (Blatterer, 2010). The most recognised markers of 'standard adulthood' (Lee, 2001), are a well-established normative model constituted through educational attainment, employment, heteronormative notions of 'making a family' and patterns of appropriate consumption. While work on contemporary transitions highlights changes in how these markers are obtained and lived, issues of how people move through the institutions of education, employment and family life remain as the key components of an adult life. They remain important norms against which young people's move into adult identities are judged and attempts to tell different narratives of what it means to be a child, adolescent or adult have been refuted. Delays in moving into stable employment still require justification; with time spent in higher education (along with a gap year of travelling overseas) still the predominant legitimate market. Therefore, those who appear to be on neither track (employment or education) become a social problem; in the UK they are often referred to as NEETs (not in employment, education, or training). Judged against the norm of successful transition, they are considered to be individually failing, rather than experiencing a precarious emerging adulthood made more difficult by shifts in employment, training possibilities and an increasingly conditional welfare system. Their failure is marked by what they so far have not achieved: individual financial and social independence. While space for experimentation may have increased, one key norm of adulthood remains, that the overarching goal should be an ability to be independent of others via one's ability to care for oneself and provide the means to do so.

Under the influence of neo-liberalism and post-industrialisation, the Global North now approaches independent adulthood as something that is the responsibility of the individual to build, prove and enact (Beck and Beck-Gernsheim, 2001; Hall et al., 1999). Clear pathways have dissolved offering up both opportunities and challenges (Bynner, 2005). For example, the pathway for young working class men in industrial locations used to be, but is no longer, school into apprenticeships, followed by the expectation of life-long employment (Willis, 1977). Nayak (2006) in an ethnography of young working class men in North-East England (the same region we do much of our research in) explored how they made sense of and developed forms of masculinity that connected them to their communities' roots in industrial labour, while working in new forms of service economy employment in low paid, part-time, temporary work environments such as call centres, shops and the leisure industry. Researchers examining young women's lives talk about both new possibilities of feminine identities that incorporate employment, education and assertiveness (Harris, 2004) and challenges of new stereotypes of femininity that continue to regulate gendered possibilities in new climates (McRobbie, 2007). The future must be made, but it also must be made to make sense in contexts where existing narratives and practices appear to no longer fit (Evans, 2002; McDowell, 2000).

Writers are beginning to make connections between the requirements to make one's own transition to adulthood to the particular body practices it may require:

> high modernity has produced an unprecedented 'individualisation' of the body, in which meanings are privatised and the body becomes a bearer of symbolic value. In consumer society it has become, in Bourdieu's terms (Bourdieu, 1984) a source of symbolic capital, less because of what the body is able to *do*, than because of how it *looks*.
>
> (original emphasis, Gill *et al.*, 2005: 40)

Individual accomplishment through care of the body is therefore an important site for regulation and validation and a measure against which people can be judged as making successful transitions. While individuality is celebrated, only certain individuals and their choices are granted approval. So there is both space to be who you want to be through your body, but only certain ways of being are then acknowledged as 'good' choices: 'the autonomous body is only allowed to make certain choices: not caring for one's physical appearance is not one of them' (Gill *et al.*, 2005: 55). Therefore for those with bodies that appear to be outside those that can embody recognised individuality there is work to do. If enacting the right kind of body projects of health, fitness, attractiveness and self-care is one way of making the right kind of individual transition, what does this mean for those whose bodies may initially be read as already in deficit by such values (Anderson, 2009)? What does this '*grammar of individualism*' (original emphasis, Gill *et al.*, 2005: 57) mean for disabled young people?

The emphasis on the individual to find their own pathway amongst expansive and new choices is problematic for the ways in which it gives less space to acknowledging socio-economic differentials, which influence people's life chances and possibilities of obtaining the kind of independence now valued as the norm (Furlong and Cartmel, 2007; White and Wyn, 2007). Prout (2000) argues that contemporary young people are working through a context that requires practices of 'self-realisation,' but does not acknowledge the ways that some people's pathways to 'independence' are supported more than others. Wyn *et al.* (2012) argue that this shift towards young people being individually responsible for providing their own pathway to an independent adult future, places greater emphasis on their family relations (rather than welfare systems) as a form of 'citizenship apparatus' (Wyn *et al.*, 2012: 10), which provides capital and support in making such pathways possible (Mørch and Andersen, 2006). The contingency and vulnerability embedded in trying to become and be an adult in a world of individualisation, means that those who are apparently able to enact independence are instead supported in multiple hidden ways (Wyn *et al.*, 2012). The difficulty then for young people, who may be living in a variety of social contexts and locations that limit the capital and resources available to them, is that the emphasis is on them to make sense of the possible futures ahead. They must find some path that seems realistic in an era where state support is minimal and visible signs of support evidence of failure (Roberts, 2011). In forming their pathway, they must also work towards a context where they appear to be self-reliant. There is then still a need to consider how socio-economic inequalities inform youth transitions, but from a perspective that includes how young people make sense of the world around and respond within their own cultural worlds (MacDonald *et al.*, 2001).

Disability is just one context highlighting that many young people have never worked through the standard model with ease. In thinking through how disabled young people respond to the complex task of becoming an adult, we need to think through how they make sense of and build narratives and practices of transition, which both incorporate shifting markers and at times provide counters to them. Across our projects both parents or carers and disabled young people have often spoken of future adulthoods, the pathways towards them and the significance of disability to what appeared possible or imaginable. A strong narrative presence within such discussions were varied ways of understanding and approaching goals of independent living.

Parental imaginaries

One of the strongest narratives from the parents or carers of disabled children we have come across is that while the present may be difficult and full of battles, it is the future they worry about most. The ways in which such fears are expressed, implies an assumption that the traditional markers of adulthood are the markers that count, and that the costs of failing to achieve them could be high. Work, having a family, living on one's own, able to manage one's own life were often rejected as impossible. Alternative or fluid ways of moving towards adulthood were few and far between. These were not contexts in which parents worried about the right university, or the risks and joys of a gap year of international travel, or the importance of young people having the time and space to 'find themselves'. Instead parents and carers were focused on standard goals of adulthood – in particular physical, economic and residential independence. Often parents or carers assumed that independence, as well as unquestionable, was also unavailable to their children as they imagined their futures:

> I know he'll, he'll always be very dependent on adult supervision, to what degree, but he'll never be independent, never be totally independent, I mean he can't even get dressed himself, and I mean, he's 8 years old, he

co-operates, sometimes he'll put his socks on, back to front or upside down, or what have you, but sometimes he'll try and do it so I mean hopefully things will settle down a bit but he'll always be dependent.

(Interview One, Harry's Mum, *Enabling Care* project)

The conflation made between independence, adulthood and normality was common amongst parents and carers. This framing is understandable. It speaks to the prevalence of such norms in how appropriate adults are recognised. It highlights a certainty of belief that differences in how one functions rule out the possibility of a future adult life that includes employment, an intimate life with others and some form of independence. Finally, it implies that once development deviates from the proper path, it will be difficult, if not impossible to find a way back. In Chapter 4 we will look at how such fears influence the push both parents and carers and young people can make to seek to repair the damage of their deviation from the appropriate path of childhood development.

The difficulty created by holding independence to be the core site of adulthood came through strongly in an interaction we had in the *Embodied Transitions* project. Lauren was considered to have learning disabilities, this led to both her mother participating in the interview and also presenting her own narrative on the difficulty Lauren would have in being independent in the way she aspired to:

INTERVIEWER: Do you have any long terms plans after college?

LAUREN: Leave home.

MUM: But she won't leave home like you've [referring to the interviewer] left home. They're going to try and get her into sheltered housing

LAUREN: No.

MUM: Well you won't be able to look after yourself.

LAUREN: No, I'm going to get a house with [boyfriend].

MUM: But you're gonna have to think, 'cos long term, Ed [the interviewer] and his friends, they manage their money, pay the bills and pay the rent, you might not be able to do that yet. You'll have to get used to that, 'cos it's hard isn't it to manage your money, pay your rent, and pay your bills?

INTERVIEWER: Well, it takes a while to learn but you've got to pick it up.

MUM: Yeah. I mean, you can just about manage money now, except for yesterday when you didn't know what things are, you have to learn to keep paying your rent every week and saving money for your bills, like your telephone bill and your electric and your gas, whatever, and your food bill. And you can do shopping 'cos you come with me all the time, don't you, so you know how to shop.

(One-Off Interview, Lauren, *Embodied Transitions* project)

There are a number of tensions around this interaction between mother, daughter and researcher (Edmund). First, it was difficult at the time to challenge the mother on the negative assessment she gave to her daughter's future ability to live independently with her boyfriend. Second, Edmund felt uncomfortable with being presented as someone who could (and by inference should) be able to handle the transition towards an independent adulthood. Third, there was a clear containment occurring over the possibilities that Lauren could form an intimate life with her boyfriend, via the likely restrictions that would be placed on where she could live as an adult and with whom. Fourth, to what degree was the mother aiding or inhibiting her daughter's possible transition towards adulthood?

Is this the classic portrayal of the over-protective parent/mother refusing her daughter's right to an independent adult future? Or was her assessment that her daughter was not ready, and potentially never could be, a reasonable assessment of what the future could be? The work done by the disability movement to promote independent living has been a vital component to significant change in disabled people's lives and something in need of protection in an era of reduced access to welfare rights. However, there is also a norm maintained in such celebration that is worth questioning. Prioritising independence leaves its status as a core marker of successful adulthood untouched. In addition, if successful independence is equated with living on your own, or in a private residential setting, other ways of living may be seen as less desirable or adult. Desiring independence or seeing its loss a tragedy helps maintain it as the ideal. It is understandable that Lauren aspires to independence, and that her mother sees it, as at least, an unlikely future. Both responses speak to the apparent unavoidability of it as a marker of adulthood to be celebrated if achieved and mourned if not. What it also led to was an apparent poverty of possible futures through which Lauren could be supported to live with her boyfriend; a poverty created by the lack of options of doing independence differently.

Parental/carer imaginaries around the future did not always stay focused on fear and loss in our research. Over time, as children grew and developed in varied ways and parents found new possibilities for their and their children's lives, imaginaries altered. Harry's mum from the *Enabling Care* project, who we quoted earlier as saying she thought her son would never be independent, in her third interview (which happened over 18 months after the first interview) spoke more positively of ways she imagined her son Harry could have a supported adult future. She could see ways that he could learn skills that would give him some independence from family, while also being provided with care and support that would enable that independence. Part of the shift people like Harry's mum made included being more willing to work with the future as unknowable. Over time, families could develop narratives of the future without fear over its uncertainty for their disabled child, or indeed what it held for their non-disabled children.

> I can sit and say well, yes what's happened to Joe is sad and I wish it hadn't had *but* because of that, you know, we've changed as a family, I've changed as a person, I've changed my job, we've moved house. We're doing things that I would have, [pause] perhaps we would never have done if we hadn't had Joe, and it's actually a lot of good come out of it. So I can be positive

about it too, I mean, it has made our lives harder, and it's made it different but in some ways it's made it better as well.

...

And, we haven't gone stupid with risk-taking behaviour and things like that but it has given us, I think a lot more freedom. Steve's packed in his job now and he's doing supply teaching and he never ever dreamed of doing that. He would have applied for deputy headships, he was on this very kind of, we were both on this kind of driven career path which we both stepped off and let go of.... I look at Cloe and think she can walk, she can talk, she's healthy, she's happy. You know, I encourage her with things but not, I don't get so worked up that she hasn't got on to the next reading book, you know at school. That some of her friends are, so what?

(Interview Two, Joe's Mum, *Enabling Care* project)

Kay's narrative provides a very different story than contained in stories of loss and tragedy. Before Joe came along the family lived within the comparatively safe world of middle class, heteronormative attainment, aspiration and living. After the diagnosis Kay had talked of wandering round IKEA in search of a sofa and feeling like she no longer belonged there. Over time this detachment from normal life was experienced as a liberation for all within the family – again validating the possibility that disabled children can be 'critical social actors' having an effect on the world around them. Disability moved Kay's family out of the norm, into a space of new possibility. This is in some ways the positive side of the era of self-actualisation: they have rejected one version of it – work hard and good things will come to you – to explore another – there are other ways to work, bring up a family and think about being and moving towards adulthood.

Being able to articulate the possibility of positive futures and alternative presents appeared more possible when childhood development was understood as more varied and open than prescribed norms can sometimes recognise. In the *Genetic Journeys* project, Charlie, the first son of Anne and Matt, had been referred to the genetics team because he had been diagnosed as being born with a key section of his brain not fully formed. The reason for that can be genetic, although during our project geneticists could not find a genetic explanation for why this had happened to Charlie. The implications of being without this part of the brain can vary significantly, with symptoms sometimes involving visual impairment, learning difficulties, seizures, speech problems and others. It is not possible to predict how the child will develop, so his mum and dad faced significant uncertainty about what the future held for Charlie. In response, after time spent trying to get a prognosis that would provide greater clarity about what the future would bring, Anne and Matt had decided to look to the future without expectation, but also with a framing that allowed for unknown possibilities as well as problems:

MUM: It has actually been kind of one of those big eye opening things where the realisation that I had him in that picket fenced house and that I was looking to the last page, I'm gonna mix several metaphors here but, had him in the picket fence house and now open to the last page of the book, and missing the rest of the journey. And what is the point in buying a novel if you just only read the last page ... I'm missing the journey, I'm missing the book, I'm not reading the book, I've decided how it's ending and that's it ... you can just enjoy him so much better ... he is different. But then who's not? Who's the same? ... that's brilliant you know. And I strongly suspect we're going to actually learn more from him than he ever learns from us.

(Interview One, Charlie's Mum and Dad, *Genetic Journeys* project)

With this freeing up of the future also came different narratives of child development that allowed in a sense of variation as within the norm:

MUM: My sister in-law hit the nail on the head when she said that before he was even born, I had him graduated from college, well university in fact, married, two kids, white picket fence, can't work the washing machine. And that reality very much in inverted commas potentially is no longer a viable proposition. I think that it's difficult for me to get my head round the fact that that might not be his reality. Or rather I *did* find it difficult because I saw I think the not-succeeding-in-job as not succeeding full-stop and my perception of the future, the way it should be with, him with a certain job, certain qualifications, certain [pause] achievements, and certain success, [pause] if he were not to achieve those I, I think I found that, that meant in my head that he wasn't gonna be successful didn't I? But over the last couple of weeks, I've got my head round the fact that success is measured in a thousand different ways. And in quite a lot of ways Charlie's already more successful than me. He makes everyone he meets smile. You know *everyone* seems to have fun with him ... Now I would love to be one of those people that instantly everybody likes, I'm not. You know, and I've always wanted to be. So, in a way, Charlie's already more successful than I am. [pause] My definition of success [speaks to Charlie] is defined by my job and as I said, we said at the beginning, being defined by your class and I think I've started to realise that I had defined his potential success by what class he would end up in and what job he would have, and what a load of rubbish.

(Interview One, Charlie's Mum and Dad, *Genetic Journeys* project)

Anne's ability to recognise that Charlie's future could be different from the norm, that his transitions to adulthood might not match the usual measures of success, led her to also recognise more broadly that such norms themselves are the problem. Other ways of being could be successful, could be valuable and may be available to her son in ways not available to her.

The contemporary narrative that the future is yours to make, also brings with it the assertion that it is parents' responsibility to ensure their children adopt that outlook on life. This story of the right kind of upbringing and future outlook can be a strong presence in how people do, or do not, make sense of imagining the future for children who seem to slip outside that category for normality. For some the monitoring nature of that norm and aspiration for the future means that thoughts for the future are filled with fear and a sense of life will always be difficult for them and their child as they grow up. Particularly, as the distance they travel from the normal transition pathways widen. Such fears are a reasonable reflection of a broader world they are already experiencing as unfriendly, unaccommodating and judgemental. However, some parents and carers appeared to have a space within which they could give up on a normal future or imagine a different normal future and embrace instead uncertainty (McLaughlin and Goodley, 2008). However, we would give one cautionary note here. In the families we have worked with who found it possible to develop approaches to uncertain futures with less fear, there was a pattern of having access to cultural and material resources, which perhaps gave them a space within which to imagine different futures, framed in the excitement of uncertainty. The space to imagine the future differently and to act upon that imaginary, is at least in part, aided by material and cultural capital.

Disabled children and young people's imaginaries

The disabled children and young people we have worked with also provide testimony to aspirations to normal futures, worries over whether they could 'make it', and glimpses of possible alternative adult imaginaries.

Disabled children and young people spoke a great deal about their preparations for adulthood, the markers they used concentred on values such as focus, determination and a concentration on planning for the future in order that they could and would succeed as adults. They appeared to believe that the future was up to them and were determined to make as much a success of themselves as possible. For example, in the *Embodied Transitions* project several spoke of career plans in ways that had moved beyond vague aspirations. Sean wished to be an airline pilot, Jamie had hoped to join the Royal Air Force; Kate was planning to go to university and train to be a medical doctor, and Jenny a veterinary nurse. All were aware that their disabilities raised challenges, but each had also researched the possibilities and were planning for their future career via the subjects they studied at school, accessing opportunities for work placements, researching their college and university options and challenging adults around them who said it would not be possible. Sean, who wished to be a pilot, had rejected an alternative career as a flight instructor and was currently challenging airlines who had no disabled pilots or adapted airplanes based on research he had done that documented cases where pilots had flown after leg amputations in conflict situations, and the modifications that would be necessary to make it possible for him to fly (not that dissimilar to the adaptations that would be made to a car).

The majority of the disabled young people in the *Embodied Transitions* project looked to the future and saw the normal markers of adulthood such as a career (not work, career) and a family as imminently possible, with just that bit of effort:

INTERVIEWER: what's your kind of image of what is a good life?

SARA: A good job, good salary, erm good friends, good family

INTERVIEWER: Yeah, what about relationships?

SARA: Yeah, maybe [laughs] good strong relationships with people yeah.

INTERVIEWER: And what about partners?

SARA: [laughs] mmm.

(One-Off Interview, Sara, *Embodied Transitions* project)

For Sara, this aspiration for a traditional version of the 'good life' was positioned against what she saw as a less desirable way of being. She spoke of a boy at her school who also had cerebral palsy. His willingness to seek help in his everyday life at school, and her assumption that he would continue to be the same as an adult, was a counter-image to her own version of growing up and becoming 'somebody':

> I'm more determined to be somebody. 'Cos if I look at him I'm thinking you will go nowhere in life because you will just let everybody do everything for you and you'll let, he's just an attention seeker.

(One-Off Interview, Sara, *Embodied Transitions* project)

The focus on these aspirations meant that disability was often positioned as something to be worked through or set aside if the young people were to live independently and be successful:

> It doesn't get in the way of what I want to do, I am ambitious and I'm not going to, it's not going to hinder us, get in the way of my ambitions and the activities that I'm doing so…. It doesn't stop us from doing anything so obviously playing football and that it doesn't stop us from doing that or it doesn't stop us from working with children. You know it might do when it comes to a job, but you know it won't make me stop wanting to work with children just because I've got cerebral palsy.

(Interview One, Rachel, *Embodied Transitions* project)

As will be returned to in Chapters 4 and 5, a narrative of disability not being a barrier to a successful transition to adulthood, was tied to intensive body practices that aimed to make disability irrelevant. It was marked how closely the young people in the *Embodied Transitions* project monitored their bodies. In particular they worked on aspects such as weight and strength through regular surveillance and acts of social control, denial and purposive building up of their muscles. Gender played its part, with strength more commonly talked of by the young men, and issues of fashion and appearance emerging more amongst the young women. However, while appearance and fashion mattered to the young women, the body was looked after, particularly in relation to weight, in order to minimise disability, rather than match feminine norms:

you can just be too skinny or you can be you know too perfect, if you know what I mean ... because I need to keep my weight down ... 'cos the surgeon say obviously 'cos my legs are weak and to keep the weight from my top half off.... Yeah so I need to try and keep slim anyway, so if I get like too heavy erm obviously my legs are weak anyway so they'll just basically collapse or stuff.... And I'll just need to use my wheelchair. So I try to keep healthy, but not too healthy, like not too slim.

(Interview One, Kate, *Embodied Transitions* project)

Kate was involved in a balancing act between norms of feminine appearance and a goal of staying mobile and out of a wheelchair (which recent surgery had enabled). Being thin was important as a marker of attractive femininity and also if she was too heavy her legs would struggle to support her and she would be back in the wheelchair. However, if she became too thin, she would lose the strength to hold up her body weight and this could also place her back in the wheelchair. Ensuring she did not become too thin or too heavy required a constant surveillance of both what she ate and what she did in terms of physical exercise. The combined effect of medical advice, norms of feminine appearance and the association of wheelchairs with a negative form of passive embodiment together produced an approach to looking after the body that emphasised the importance of self-discipline to become a valued young woman.

It is hard to escape the current importance being given to individual healthy living in public health regulation (Lupton, 1995). This was a message found often in the narratives young people in the *Embodied Transitions* project used to explain how they looked after their body:

INTERVIEWER: So what do you do to manage your weight then?
LAUREN: Eat healthy. Exercise, eat fruit, go to the gym on a Wednesday.
INTERVIEWER: What kind of stuff do you do at the gym?
LAUREN: I go on the exercise bike, the walker [treadmill], the pedal bike, and the boat [rowing machine].

(One-Off Interview, Lauren, *Embodied Transitions* project)

Living well, was a constant imperative, one that required constant monitoring to ensure no slip ups in improvement and control:

I have to remind myself though to exercise my arm. If I forget to exercise it then it kind of 'creeps up'.

(One-Off Interview, Jamie, *Embodied Transitions* project)

Disabled young people asserting that such future career pathways are imaginable and attainable (with personal effort and determination) implies a contemporary setting in which transitions to positive adult futures are not incompatible with disability. They are aware of legislative change that means (in theory) that people cannot simply reject someone for being disabled. They could be a pilot, or a veterinary nurse, or a medical doctor and be disabled. One element of making varied futures possible, outside prescribed pathways, is that who is imagined to be present within such futures is opened up to broader categories of people. This in itself implies an expansion of the possible transitions to adulthood as a part of contemporary disabled young people's lives.

Nevertheless we hesitate over suggesting this contemporary landscape is unconditionally a good thing. This hesitation is over potential costs that come with this contemporary landscape for disabled young people imagining and striving towards their adult futures. The disabled young people we worked with in the *Embodied Transitions* project had, for the most part, mind-body differences that were not as significant as others can have. For those with differences further from societal norms of how minds-bodies function there was less evidence of the opening up of adult imaginaries that others thought realisable. Amongst those in the project with the most significant mismatch between how the world is ordered and their minds-bodies functioned, there was greater scepticism about what the future held and whether they would be able to do things like find a job (a job rather than a career), or leave the family home. This means that heightened hierarchies maybe developing between those disabled young people able (as much through the capital available to them as their own personal effort) to make successful transitions and those judged to either not have the capacity or have failed in their attempt to reach it. We are reminded of Sara's clear distain for her fellow disabled pupil who she believed was not trying hard enough. The possibility that disabled young people can succeed as a norm can become a pressure to succeed, and for those who do not get on in the ways proscribed, the fault can appear to lie with them. The new possibilities emerging for disabled young people are occurring alongside long term patterns of precarious welfare rights and economic insecurity. This means that access to resources and capital will continue to be important to the realisation of such possibilities, generating significant inequalities in the transitions disabled young people will make (Wyn *et al.*, 2012).

Because structures of inequality and marginalisation are made less visible in narratives of self-realisation, it appears there is less recognition that the future is not just made, it can also be made impossible by social conditions not of the individual's making. Earlier, Rachel asserted strongly that disability would not be a barrier to her life being what she wanted to make it. However, in her second interview, she spoke of the difficulties she was having finding a job. Currently she was doing voluntary work in a shop because so far she had been unable to find employment in the area she would like: working with children. Difficulties getting even part time jobs while at school were not uncommon amongst the young people in our research. As part of her cerebral palsy, Rachel had mild epileptic seizures, while she had been told this should not be a barrier to working with children, she believed that schools would prefer to have someone who did not have the condition. No matter how hard Rachel works, the prejudicial actions of others will still affect her life chances.

What all this means is that whilst the range of people who may gain a successful adulthood may have broadened, what defines that adulthood appears not to have. In particular independence remains a central norm of adulthood disabled young people aspire to:

SARA: I'm a lot more independent now, so it's quite alright for me now, whereas before it just I'd just I'd rely on my mum and my dad to make choices and stuff for me. But now I'm getting to the age where I can fend for myself, if you know what I mean? Slightly more than I would. So I'm getting more independent.

INTERVIEWER: And what do you mean by that?

SARA: Just go out on my own, with friends. Do my own thing.

(One-Off Interview, Sara, *Embodied Transitions* project)

Disability writers have tried to broaden out societal narratives of what independence can contain. They have both challenged the degree to which anyone is 'truly' independent, and argued that if a personal assistant enables someone to live on their own by helping them wash, dress, cook, look after their home, then they have facilitated independent living. Disabled young people were aware and open to some of the contingencies of independent living and included access to support in their plans for future independence:

I do eventually want to move out when I'm eighteen but it's getting the help, I don't know what help is out there to help me do that [pause]. I mean don't get me wrong there's probably money or something out there that's available when I'm eighteen to get me own place but it's finding a place that's accessible, no steps or anything for me to move into, and able to keep tidy by myself, I personally don't need twenty four hour care, I might need somebody to come in and help read, read me bills, come in and help me put me socks and boots on, go around with the hoover. Other than that I'm totally independent.

(One-Off Interview, Ryan, *Embodied Transitions* project)

Nevertheless where possible what the disabled young people wanted to do was to do things and achieve things by and for themselves as the true marker of independence:

MARK: You'd rather be doing things for yourself rather than people be doing things for you or, I know I would. I'd rather be independent than trying to get people to wait on me hand and foot, it might take ten minutes extra but if you're doing it yourself for ten minutes, what's ten minutes if you're doing it yourself rather than somebody that'd take five if you did it yourself it takes ten, take ten and do it yourself than take five take whatever to get someone else to do it for you.

INTERVIEWER: So do you think being independent, how important is independence?

MARK: Oh it's huge it's I would say it's [under] rated sometimes I think it's absolutely massive to do things for yourself, it gives you that sense of quite often, well carrying a bag in my eyes it's quite a good thing 'cos it's just you, it might fall off your lap three or four times but you get there in the end and yeah just things like that give you a little, little buzz. It might not be much but carrying a bag or carrying a pint back you know, carrying a drink back with having to use your hands to push it's like, obviously it's quite good and to do things yourself is a lot better than getting other people to do it for you is massive. My independence is a lot yeah. Doing things yourself is overrated, underrated sorry.

(Interview One, Mark, *Embodied Transitions* project)

Transitions to adulthood are changing for disabled children and young people, as they are for others. On one level they offer opportunities for greater participation in normal adult life than has been possible in the past. On another, there is evidence of fragility, inequality and cost within these shifting transitions, as the requirement to successfully transition across a relatively unchanging goal of individual independence remains unchanged.

Conclusion

Disabled children and young people are now present in many mainstream school environments, there are now expectations that they will also grow up to be adult participants in society. The normal has expanded to include them. However, concepts of what is normal continue to have a disciplinary power that serves to exclude and segregate within the institutions of mainstream society. Across school and transitions to adulthood the work of accommodating to existing norms falls on the disabled child and young person. If they seem unable to reach such accommodations the fault is said to be theirs. The social privileges and capital that some have access to, which can help them succeed within existing norms is not given adequate recognition. As the legitimacy and scope of welfare support further declines, the risk is that the gap between those who can succeed and those who cannot will grow and the penalties for being in the group who did not succeed will become even higher. What this chapter has also made visible is the need to continue to challenge on the policing qualities of normative assumptions about the 'normal' way of being a child and an adult. This includes the ways we value and think about independence. Chapter 7 will return to this theme by exploring the relationship between values of independence with recognition of the productive citizen.

References

Anderson, D. (2009) Adolescent girls' involvement in disability sport: implications for identity development. *Journal of Sport & Social Issues*, 33(4): 427–449.
Arnett, J.J. (2004) *Emerging Adulthood: The Winding Road from the Late Teens through the Twenties*. Oxford: Oxford University Press.

Ashby, C. (2010) The trouble with normal: the struggle for meaningful access for middle school students with developmental disability labels. *Disability & Society*, 25(3): 345–358.

Beck, U. and Beck-Gernsheim, E. (2001) *Individualization: Institutionalized Individualism and Its Social and Political Consequences*. London: Sage.

Blatterer, H. (2010) The changing semantics of youth and adulthood. *Cultural Sociology*, 4(1): 63–79.

Bourdieu, P. (1984) *Distinction: A Social Critique of the Judgement of Taste*. London: Routledge.

Bradley, H. and Devadason, R. (2008) Fractured transitions: young adults' pathways into contemporary labour markets. *Sociology*, 42(1): 119–136.

Bynner, J.M. (2005) Rethinking the youth phase of the life-course: the case for emerging adulthood? *Journal of Youth Studies*, 8(4): 367–384.

Clark, S., Kabiru, C. and Mathur, R. (2010) Relationship transitions among youth in urban Kenya. *Journal of Marriage and Family*, 72(1): 73–88.

Coles, B. (2000) *Joined up Youth Research, Policy and Practice*. Leicester: Youth Work Press.

Davis, J.M. and Watson, N. (2001) Where are the children's experiences? Analysing social and cultural exclusion in 'special' and 'mainstream' schools. *Disability & Society*, 16(5): 671–687.

Dwyer, P. and Wyn, J. (2001) *Youth, Education and Risk: Facing the Future*. London: Routledge.

Evans, K. (2002) Taking control of their lives? Agency in young adult transitions in England and the new Germany. *Journal of Youth Studies*, 5(3): 245–269.

Foucault, M. (1990) *The History of Sexuality Volume 1: An Introduction*. New York, NY: Vintage Books.

Foucault, M. (1991) Governmentality. In G. Burchell, C. Gordon and P. Miller (eds), *The Foucault Effect: Studies in Governmentality*. pp. 87–104. London: Harvester/Wheatsheaf.

Furlong, A. and Cartmel, F. (2007) *Young People and Social Change*. New York, NY: Open University Press.

Furlong, A., Woodman, D. and Wyn, J. (2011) Changing times, changing perspectives: reconciling 'transition' and 'cultural' perspectives on youth and young adulthood. *Journal of Sociology*, 47(4): 355–370.

Gardner, H. (1993) *Multiple Intelligences: The Theory in Practice* New York, NY: Basic Books.

Gill, R., Henwood, K. and McLean, C. (2005) Body projects and the regulation of normative masculinity. *Body & Society*, 11: 37–62.

Gillies, V. (2000) Young people and family life: analysing and comparing disciplinary discourses. *Journal of Youth Studies*, 3(2): 18–26.

Grant, M.J. and Furstenberg, F.F. (2007) Changes in the transition to adulthood in less developed countries. *European Journal of Population*, 23: 415–428.

Hall, T., Coffey, A. and Williamson, H. (1999) Self, space and place: youth identities and citizenship. *British Journal of Sociology of Education*, 20(4): 501–513.

Harris, A. (2004) Young Australian women: circumstances and aspirations. *Youth Studies Australia*, 21(4): 32–37.

Harry, B. and Kalyanpur, M. (1994) Cultural underpinnings of special education: implications for professional interactions with culturally diverse families. *Disability & Society*, 9(2): 145–165.

Holdsworth, C., and Morgan, D. (2005) *Transitions in Context: Leaving Home, Independence and Adulthood.* Maidenhead: Open University Press.

Holloway, S.L. and Valentine, G. (2000) Spatiality and the new social studies of childhood. *Sociology*, 34: 763–783.

Holt, L. (2004a) Children with mind-body differences: performing disability in primary school classrooms. *Children's Geographies*, 2(2): 219–236.

Holt, L. (2004b) Childhood disability and ability: (dis)ableist geographies of mainstream primary schools. *Disability Studies Quarterly*, 24(3).

Holt, L., Bowlby, S. and Lea, J. (2013) Emotions and the habitus: young people with socio-emotional differences (re)producing social, emotional and cultural capital in family and leisure space-times. *Emotion, Space and Society*, 9(Nov): 33–41.

Holt, L., Lea, J. and Bowlby, S. (2012) Special units for young people on the autistic spectrum in mainstream schools: sites of normalisation, abnormalisation, inclusion, and exclusion. *Environment and Planning A*, 44: 2191–2206.

Honneth, A. (1996) *The Struggle for Recognition: The Moral Grammar of Social Conflict.* Cambridge: Polity Press.

Imrie, R. (2013) Shared space and the post-politics of environmental change. *Urban Studies*, 50(16): 3446–3462.

Jones, G., O'Sullivan, A. and Rouse, J. (2006) Young adults, partners and parents: individual agency and the problems of support. *Journal of Youth Studies*, 9(4): 375–392.

Kittay, E.F. (2006) Thoughts on the desire for normality. In E. Parens (ed.), *Surgically Shaping Children: Technology, Ethics and the Pursuit of Normality.* pp. 90–110. Baltimore, MD: The Johns Hopkins University Press.

Lee, N. (2001) *Childhood and Society.* Buckingham: Open University Press.

Lupton, D. (1995) *The Imperative of Health.* London: Sage.

MacDonald, R. (2011) Youth transitions, unemployment and underemployment. *Journal of Sociology*, 17(1): 127 141.

MacDonald, R., Mason, P., Shildrick, T., Webster, C., Johnston, L. and Ridley, L. (2001) Snakes & ladders: in defence of studies of youth transition. *Sociological Research Online*, 5(4): http://socresonline.org.uk/5/4/macdonald.html

Madriaga, M., Hanson, K., Kay, H. and Walker, A. (2011) Marking-out normalcy and disability in higher education. *British Journal of Sociology of Education*, 32(6): 901–920.

McDowell, L. (2000) Learning to serve? Employment aspirations and attitudes of young working-class men in an era of labour market restructuring *Gender, Place and Culture*, 7(4): 389–416.

McLaughlin, J. and Goodley, D. (2008) Seeking and rejecting certainty: exposing the sophisticated lifeworlds of parents of disabled babies. *Sociology*, 42(2): 317–335.

McRobbie, A. (2007) Top girls? Young women and the post-feminist sexual contract. *Cultural Studies*, 21(4–5): 718–737.

Moola, F.J. and Norman, M.E. (2011) 'Down the rabbit hole': enhancing the transition process for youth with cystic fibrosis and congenital heart disease by re-imagining the future and time. *Child: Care Health and Development*, 37(6): 841–851.

Mørch, S. and Andersen, H. (2006) Individualization and the changing youth life. In C. Leccardi and E. Ruspini (eds), *A New Youth? Young People, Generations and Family Life.* pp. 63–84. Aldershot: Ashgate.

Nadesan, M.H. (2005) *Constructing Autism: Unraveling the 'Truth' and Understanding the Social.* New York, NY: Routledge.

Naraian, S. and Natarajan, P. (2013) Negotiating normalcy with peers in contexts of inclusion: perceptions of youth with disabilities in India. *International Journal of Disability Development and Education*, 60(2): 146–166.

Nayak, A. (2006) Displaced masculinities: chavs, youth and class in the post-industrial city. *Sociology*, 40(5): 813–831.

Olin, E. and Jansson, B.R. (2009) On the outskirts of normality: young adults with disabilities, their belonging and strategies. *International Journal of Qualitative Studies on Health and Well-Being*, 4(4): 256–266.

Prout, A. (2000) Children's participation: control and self-realisation in British late modernity. *Children & Society*, 14(4): 304–315.

Rao, S. (2001) 'A little inconvenience': perspectives of Bengali families of children with disabilities on labelling and inclusion. *Disability & Society*, 16(4): 531–548.

Roberts, S. (2011) Beyond 'NEET' and 'tidy' pathways: considering the 'missing middle' of youth transition studies. *Journal of Youth Studies*, 14(1): 21–39.

Rogers, R. (2011) 'I remember thinking, why isn't there someone to help me? Why isn't there someone who can help me make sense of what I'm going through?' 'Instant adulthood' and the transition of young people out of state care. *Journal of Sociology*, 47(4): 411–426.

Vlachou, A.D. (1997) *Struggles for Inclusion: An Ethnographic Study*. Buckingham: Open University Press.

Warner, M. (1999) *The Trouble with Normal: Sex, Politics, and the Ethics of Queer Life*. Cambridge, MA: Harvard University Press.

White, R. and Wyn, J. (2007) *Youth and Society: Exploring the Social Dynamics of Youth Experience*. Oxford: Oxford University Press.

Wierenga, A. (2011) Transitions, local culture and human dignity: rural young men in a changing world. *Journal of Sociology*, 47(4): 371–387.

Willis, P. (1977) *Learning to Labour: How Working Class Kids Get Working Class Jobs*. London: Saxon House.

Winzer, M.A. (1993) *The History of Special Education: From Isolation to Integration*. Washington, DC: Gallaudet University Press.

Worth, N. (2009) Understanding youth transition as 'becoming': identity, time and futurity. *Geoforum*, 40(6): 1050–1060.

Wyn, J., Lantz, S. and Harris, A. (2012) Beyond the 'transitions' metaphor: family relations and young people in late modernity. *Journal of Sociology*, 48(1): 3–22.

4 Engagements with medical diagnosis and intervention

Medical sociology (Stiker, 2000) and disability studies (Barnes and Mercer, 2010; Illich, 1976) have both detailed medicine's authority in informing the belief that certain body types and persons fall outside measures of normality, categorising 'different' bodies as disabled and undesirable and offering up treatments for their difference. Foucault (1975, [1976] 1990) meticulously highlighted the politics of and processes involved in the establishment of 'normal bodies' through medicine's categorisation of bodies considered outside of the normal. Those drawing from his ideas (Conrad, 1992; Conrad and Schneider, 1980; Feder, 2008) use them to show how medicine has done more than identify and help us understand the sources of normal and abnormal function and capacity. Instead it has been productive in shaping the types of bodies drawn into the protection of being defined as 'normal' and those positioned as abnormal and in need of treatment (Hoffman, 2013). In doing so, as Davis (1995: 30) has famously argued, medicine produced the 'concept of the disabled body' Embodied difference in childhood has always been a particular fascination within such productive practices, particularly differences that have taken children away from expected pathways of development.

More recently, the concept of medicalisation has undergone conceptual scrutiny. An important aspect has been to ask does the passive acceptance of medical categories and power, which some versions of it imply, match the ways in which people now engage with medicine? Can medicine as an institution dictate the boundaries of human acceptability and normality? Patient advocacy groups, through both fundraising and political campaigning, now play an important part in shaping medical agendas; including in medical research focused on childhood disability. While many operate within medical priorities of cure and treatment, they nevertheless broaden the constituency of voices influencing medical practice. The disability movement and third sector groups focused on political and social agendas now challenge the supremacy of medical responses to disability and call for greater social inclusion and action instead. The spread of communication and information technologies enable patients, or their parents/guardians, to come to medicine with their own knowledge and understanding of their bodies. Medical expertise may resist attempts by patients or others to interpret and diagnose based on their own research, but the notion that the 'doctor knows best' and is unchallengeable is dwindling; helped by public accounts of both medical mistakes and malpractice. We are also being asked to be participants in our health; whether this is as the consumers of neo-liberal accounts (Newman and Vidler, 2006), or the expert patient of biocitizen-ship (Rose and Novas, 2005), we are supposed to be active in looking after our health and responding to our bodily frailties.

In response writers examining the influence and power of medicine from a variety of disciplinary perspectives have sought to find new or altered ways to understand the scope and form of its social significance. Critical disability studies has been important through the emphasis it gives to language and cat-egorisation as something that both secures medical power, as well as something which can be countered via different linguistic imaginaries to reflect varied human possibilities (Shildrick, 2005). Alongside, we find contemporary fem-inist work on science and medicine particularly useful given its consideration of both the productive power of medicine and the broader landscapes of meaning and social interaction it sits within (Braidotti, 2002; Clarke and Fujimura, 1992; Haraway, 1991). This work acknowledges that innovations in areas such as pharmaceuticals (Asberg and Johnson, 2009) and neurosciences (Wilson, 2004) have the 'power to define appropriate humanness' (Asberg and Lum, 2009: 333). But it also explores how such technologies can become significant cultural artefacts incorporated into the personhood practices of women and others (Draper, 2002; Nishizaka, 2011). It pauses to consider what people do with medical technologies and practices and how they develop meaning through them.

For example, ultrasound scanning in pregnancy has a long history of feminist analyses. This work has critiqued it as something that objectifies the pregnant body and wrestles knowledge of the pregnancy from the woman and her embod-ied experience and places it on the screen and in the medical gaze of the 'expert' interpreting the image held there (Birke, 1999; Petchesky, 1987; Zechmeister, 2001). Contemporary feminist work on ultrasound, while acknowledging that it contains these dangers, by studying the interactions women have with the tech-nology and the meaning they give to it, also include the significance of that inter-action in what emerges. Roberts argues, in an ethnographic study of the growth of 4D commercial ultrasound scanning, that future parents are active in creating meaning from the technology through the ways in which they are 'mobilising family knowledge and embodied experience in order to narrate the imagery on the screen in a way that is both socially and personally meaningful' (Roberts, 2012: 299–300). Similarly, in an analysis of paediatric genetics, Latimer (2013) refers to 'relations of exchange' that occur between the multiple actors and arte-facts. She proposes that each actor present in the diagnostic encounter brings something to it that shapes what occurs and what meanings will emerge from it for both child under scrutiny and their wider family. In the context of genetics, medicine and kinship come together to create narratives through which both the child and differences in development are framed and understood. The notion of exchange does not rule out the possibility that there may be inequalities of resource or authority in such exchanges, but does allow us to consider that medical actors are not the only ones who will have a say in defining the significances to be drawn from what the expert 'sees'.

We find contemporary feminist approaches to conceptualising medicine's influence on shaping understandings of disabled childhoods particularly useful for two reasons. First, it enables us to populate the institution of medicine with the interactions that occur within it (Mol, 2002). As an institution still given significant value and status in society, medicine has a privileged position in setting the rules of its practice and influence through the claims to knowledge and expertise it maintains, its ability to frame the categories through which bodies are understood, and to advocate for the treatment options it pursues. However, how people interact with those rules and practices influences both the immediate outcomes for a particular patient and the people around them and more broadly can influence the status of medicine itself. In the interactions between patients, those close to them, and the range of medical actors they can encounter, a broader range of meanings, understandings and practices come to shape what emerges from those interactions. Second, this feminist approach encourages the researcher to move out from the clinic into the everyday contexts of people's broader lives and relationships. If we start with medicine we presume it is the leading institution framing our modes of understanding human life. When a child enters the world of medicine they are already within a set of relationships and narratives influencing their understanding of themselves and other's understandings of them. Medicine will be drawn into those pre-existing understandings through both language and embodied practice. Therefore, our interest lies in understanding both the interactions and the broader landscapes of meaning that influence how people engage with each other and medicine; including the children themselves.

Our focus remains on the role of medicine in defining the boundaries of human acceptability. As we have already discussed an important activity disabled children and young people are involved in is their management of the responses of others to the ways in which their bodies, minds, behaviours may differ. We are interested in how medicine both influences such management and is also influenced by such management. Overall, the chapter seeks to engage with how medicine participates in problematic practices of normalisation, but also to explore ways in which we may understand that dynamic more fully, including disabled children and young people's own involvement both in conforming to normalisation and also challenging it. The chapter is structured around a focus on two core aspects of medical practice: diagnosis and intervention.

Diagnosis

Our most concentrated exploration of diagnosis was within the *Genetic Journeys* project. A focus on genetics was not a random choice. Within contemporary medicine genetics is an increasing presence within diagnostic practices – particularly for children with unusual development. This has been fuelled by advances in genetic techniques, which promise that the day when our whole genome will be mapped at birth (or before) is now not far from our – or medicine's – grasp. Such mapping will identify patterns of genetic variation not seen before and (over time) link more of those variations to named and medically validated disorders. Differences in child development lie at the centre of much of the research ongoing (for example the Deciphering Developmental Disorders (DDD) study run from the Wellcome Trust Sanger Institute in the UK); one of the things such research promises is to give a 'name' and in the future a prognosis to children who currently have no clear explanation or illness category for their differences in development. Such knowledge is presumed to be a good thing that brings benefits (such as ending the uncertainty and lack of clarity over why a child is different and what the future may bring) to the child and their carers. Such developments could mean that complex analyses of blood will become more important to diagnosis, rather than examinations of the child's body and the differences they display (the current starting point of new referrals to paediatric genetics). At the time of our study physical examinations of the child's body remained an important aspect of the diagnostic process, however some of the newer techniques that allow visual display of smaller fragments of DNA via complex computational calculations, were beginning to be used and drawn into consultations we observed. This provides an avenue to think about whether the relational body and the interactions and narratives around it, remain in some way present and meaningful in the way Roberts (2012) argues is still the case within 4D ultrasound scanning.

Some medical sociologists argue that genetics is a new form of medical gaze, which no longer requires symptoms or a body in order to delineate between different kinds of person and to produce the disabled body (Featherstone *et al.*, 2005; Novas and Rose, 2000). As evidence they point to medical statements such as the editorial in the *New England Journal of Medicine* that predicted 'Clinicians, like researchers, can now shift to a 'genotype first' model of diagnosis for children with unexplained developmental abnormalities' (Ledbetter, 2008: 1729–1730). The implication is that chromosomal differences represented in computer diagrams are 'the essential referent of new categories of illness' (Navon, 2011: 204). Buchbinder and Timmermans (2011: 57) argue that you can see this shift occurring in the growing scope of neonatal genetic screening in the US. Here the screening technologies and the molecular disorders being investigated are so new that what is being identified are 'ontologically disputed borderline forms of disease' and understandings of child development. For Bleakley and Bligh (2009), influenced by Baudrillard (1994), the use of such technologies symbolises a shift in the operation of medical power, as the ability to produce and interpret a simulation of the body becomes the ground upon which medical power and authority plays out. What this could imply is that medicalisation is finding a new outlet via the virtual, where its versions of difference are feeding into contemporary 'body-world relations, and ideas of personhood, identity and belonging' (Latimer, 2013: 7).

Such possibilities are undeniable, however, in considering them we need to bear in mind the shifting ways in which medicalisation is now being understood. In particular, we wish to take the broader context of relational embodiment and social landscapes into consideration (Hoffman, 2013). The benefit of doing so is that it helps us think through how the body may still be significant to the relations of exchange such diagrams and images become part of. Giving the diagram the power to delineate forms of acceptable and unacceptable personhood risks seeing what happens in the clinic as being the only factor of significance. It narrows the clinical dynamic down to laboratory processes that occur away from the patient and their broader world. As Mol (2002: 24) notes '…what is needed, indeed indispensable for clinical diagnosis, is that there be a patient-body'. The geneticist cannot go very far without a body and that body does not exist purely in the laboratory or consultation room. By reflecting on the multiple ways the body was significant to relations of exchange within the diagnostic processes we studied in the *Genetic Journeys* project, we aim to highlight how, even in the increasingly virtual realm of genetics, the body still matters. It matters not just as something medicine seeks to define, but as something with significant social and cultural meaning and value that others shape.

Gazing upon the body

Even as genetics increasingly turns to complex biochemical analyses and computer generated visualisations of chromosomes to identify genetic variation, it still must come in contact with the child. Not least because, outside of screening programmes, it is differences in the development of a child's body that does not look, or move, or interact with the world in the way it 'should' that leads to her being seen by paediatric genetics in the first place. It is important to remain curious about what occurs within such encounters; as it points to the relational quality of the embodied interactions that occur there, which are then followed through into the encounters with diagrams of DNA. Our observations in the *Genetic Journeys* project included many first consultations that focused on micro examinations of the child's body by the geneticist (McLaughlin and Clavering, 2012).

> Geneticist comes down onto honkers, at eye-level with Jake, who puts his head down…
>
> At this point the geneticist's tone of voice is very soft, very slow and gentle, speaking to Jake: Can I see your hand too? Thank you very much.
>
> Still speaking in very gentle tone, the geneticist nods to the mother and asks: And you are seeing Dr [X], and you think his eyes are ok?
>
> While speaking, the focus of the geneticist's gaze remains on Jake all the time.
>
> Mother: They're fine, though he has got a lazy eye…
>
> Geneticist stands back up: Can we just pop his top off?
>
> Once the mother removes child's top, the geneticist asks Jake in very upbeat but still gentle tone: Can I just hold you for one minute?

Geneticist then looks at the mother: It's just to get a sense of his weight, and his body … You're quite a floppy boy.

(Observation notes of first consultation, Jake, Mum, Dad, Geneticist and Paediatrician, *Genetic Journeys* project)

Consultants described this process to us and to parents and children as about 'looking for clues'. Such close examinations placed the child's body under intense scrutiny; the focus was on identifying why she or he looked different from the norm. In doing so distinctive physical characteristics moved from being visible but benign variations, to being markers of potential genetic otherness. This kind of close physical examination emphasises the peculiarity of a child's body and dissects the child into an object of micro-medical scrutiny:

She [the daughter] was a bit of meat on the bed. The geneticist was doing their job; I don't have any resentment about that. But it just became, she became like an object. It was very, it just felt clinical and I didn't like it. The geneticist was looking at bits of her.

(Interview One, Alesha's Mum, *Genetic Journeys* project)

These dynamics would appear to be textbook examples of producing a medicalised body, one narrowed to what medicine finds of interest in quests to find disorder. However, in thinking through the full significance of medicine's reading of the child's body we also need to consider how the parents, others and the child place that reading in their broader landscapes of meaning and identity. When parents discussed the scrutiny their child received, it was clear that medicine was not the only source of meaning that influenced their reading of their child as a consequence of that scrutiny. In particular, and no surprise since genetics is the context here, ties of kinship were important networks of meaning and location through which children and their embodiment were read. When a child is investigated for having some form of genetic variation, it carries the risk of distorting the kinship bonds the child is within (Edwards, 2005; Featherstone *et al.*, 2006). Either it suggests that the kinship line contains an existing fault, or the child has introduced a fault into the line (a *de novo* mutation). Due to the importance of kinship to belonging and identity, medicine may be involved in drawing that difference to the forefront, but it is within existing narratives of kinship that sense will be made of that difference (Strathern, 1992).

For example, alongside the examination of the child's body, geneticists spend a significant aspect of the first consultation exploring the family tree of the child's extended family. The way in which the tree is developed is shaped by the possibilities the geneticists are considering for explaining the child's differences in development. In particular, they pay more attention to the paternal or maternal line depending on which side is associated with specific types of genetic variation under consideration. The genetic variation geneticists thought Sophie may have had was linked to the maternal line; this led them to focus their mapping out of the family tree to that side. Sophie's biological dad reacted strongly to the lack of interest in his side of the family tree:

DAD: They did like a little family tree of like how many brothers and sisters her mother had got, and her [maternal] grandmother had got, and ages and all that … I said to you [mum] I was getting annoyed, 'cos they only did you two [mum and grandmother], they didn't actually ask any questions about my family and my brother's and sister's heights and that. But you said it is just because it was your genes…

MUM: Because it comes from me, so they wanted to know my family history and things like that.

INTERVIEWER [TO DAD]: When you say annoyed, why did you feel annoyed, if you don't mind me asking?

DAD: Well they was doing their family tree, I wasn't even on it.

(Interview One, Sophie's Mum, Dad and Grandmother,
Genetic Journeys project)

The drawing of the tree without the father's presence implied that his biological relationship to his daughter was of less significance than that of the mother and her side of the family. He was aware of the medical basis for this emphasis, but that was not necessarily enough to reassure him. This was because this feeling of detachment was not just a product of genetics. As Strathern (1992) points out, paternity is the easiest connection to erase given the significance of the mother's body to pregnancy and birth. Paternity is something that has to be made visible. The sense of erasure the father spoke of was connected to an existing dislocation he felt by being from another part of the country and therefore an incomer to an existing located kinship group. At various points in interviews with us Sophie's dad described himself as a 'foreigner' because he was not from the North of England, genetics then adds to this broader narrative of 'non-belonging' by not including him in the family tree.

The social and biological came together to imply his presence within the family was less rooted and less important to the child's character and future. For this reason he worked to remake the connection to his child. One visual symbol of the trait that Sophie was being considered for is short stature. In the interview her dad commented, 'I mean I am not the tallest of people'. While the genetics consultant asserted that her stature was related to the trait that can only be passed on by the mother, the father found a way to bring himself back into the explanation via the shared embodied characteristic he saw and could narrate. The father's sense of distance from the family and his route back in is through a relational practice that draws from medicine, but also from social and intimate ties of connection that the genetic interest in the family tree as a representation of family could not break.

The presence of a child's body in the clinical encounter brings the broader meanings, in this case kinship, already shaping her identity by others into that encounter. It influences how people respond to clinical interpretations of what the body represents and shapes the way they seek to protect those meanings from the potential encroachment genetics can bring as it reinterprets and repositions kinship ties. This is something we will return to in Chapter 6. This part has focused on interactions where the body is present; what happens when the process moves away from the body, towards the diagram?

Gazing at the diagram

In the *Genetic Journeys* project we observed several consultations where a clear shift occurred from examinations of the child's body, to examination and fascination with computer diagrams of chromosomal variation. Below is a typical observational extract highlighting how a geneticist described a diagram they had produced of genetic sequencing of a particular section of a chromosome:

> Geneticist returns to the diagrams ... 'So, if we look here [pointing] you can see [numbered chromosome] is in the right place, where the red blob is, [numbered chromosome] is also in the right place, but one has ended up on chromosome [number]. So we had a close look at that. Chromosome [number] had a normal look to it, but here there is a bit of chromosome [number] on [numbered chromosome].'
>
> (Observation notes of second consultation, Alesha, Mum, Dad and Geneticist, *Genetic Journeys* project)

Parents often were impressed by what the diagrams were able to display, Grace's father was amazed by how they could capture such tiny variations within his daughter's DNA:

> He [the consultant] drew a diagram and he said there's like a bar code, you know how they put a bar code on the back of a cornflake box or something? And it's one, it's like one little line and it has like millions and millions of little chromosomes inside that do different things, and it's one of them that's missing.
>
> (Interview Two, Grace's Mum and Dad, *Genetic Journeys* project)

Grace had been provided with a diagnosis that said she was missing material from a specific chromosome. In their second interview her mum and dad discussed how they had been fascinated by this finding and its display for some time – including jokingly calling Grace 'Chromo 12' – for a time. However, their fascination was limited by how little they discovered the diagram could actually say about Grace. During the consultation, after going into great detail about how they had been able to produce the diagram, the consultant admitted that due to the newness of the technology there was little they could deduce about Grace's future. Indeed he acknowledged the finding could be a 'red herring' and have little to do with the issues she faced. Grace's mum and dad found this very frustrating; particularly because they had been called in to hear about findings – for them dots on a diagram were not a finding:

DAD: I think, because we thought we were going to go and they could tell us everything we wanted to know, but they didn't tell us anything, because they didn't know.

...

MUM: in the letter it said, 'when you come for this appointment, as well as the blood test, we'll discuss in detail'

...

DAD: So I thought 'the detail' meant the outlook, but it wasn't, it was the detail about how they did it, how they got to this stage.

(Interview Two, Grace's Mum and Dad, *Genetic Journeys* project)

This pattern of interaction and disappointment was common as parents tried to find out what the diagrams could meaningfully say about the future for their children:

GENETICIST: 'She has a pattern, what we call a Mosaic. This is where people have different pictures in different cells, rather than a single cell being affected. I can't say she won't be having more problems in the future, but what I can say is that, in other cases with similar chromosome patterns, none of them have presented with the same problems. So you should treat her as entirely unique. We will need to keep her under review, to see how she goes'.

Geneticist looks at Alesha's mum and smiles, then looks back down to the page, pointing with a pen, and then up to her dad.

GENETICIST: 'I'm sorry I can't tell you about what to expect at this stage'.

(Observation notes of second consultation, Alesha, Mum, Dad and Geneticist, *Genetic Journeys* project)

The limited explanation the medical interpretation of the diagram can provide reduces the exchange value it can sustain. As it travels further into the familial world of the child the exchange possibilities continue but – as we shall see – they remain contained. After consultations where 'findings' were discussed families would receive letters detailing the test that had been undertaken, the geneticist's interpretation (often one to two pages of medical explanation), and a copy of the diagram displaying the genetic variation found. It is not unusual for parents of disabled or ill children to meticulously collate and store such medical documents. The way they are looked after, displayed and annotated often alongside other artefacts, such as photographs relating to the child, integrates them into the relational world of the family. What this means is that the meaning of the letters is produced alongside other artefacts and other remembrances of family ties. Alesha's mum treated the letter she received explaining what they had found with a significant level of respect. She wanted to know more about what it meant and sought further medical explanation to help her understand it:

MUM: We got the letter after the last consultation at genetics, and we can see Alesha's situation is complicated – her chromosome disorder is very complex. It was very difficult to take it all in. I called the geneticist a couple of times after the consultation to ask questions, and went on the internet to try and make sense of what it will all mean for Alesha over time. What the geneticist told us was that Alesha's chromosome disorder is unique to her. She has a balanced translocation, where some of her Chromosome [N] and [N] have swapped over. But also she has a bit of Chromosome [N] missing – what they call a deletion. This is all connected with her medical problems – the difficulties she has are because of her chromosome disorder/translocation.

(Second Interview, Alesha's Mum and Aunt, *Genetic Journeys* project)

A relation of exchange had occurred here, the letter provided something the mother wanted – a possible explanation for why her child was the way she was – in return she treated it with authority and curiosity. As the discussion carried on, Alesha's mum picked up the letter and pointed to the diagram showing the chromosome variation and said:

This is Alesha, this is Alesha really, it is her, she is unique.

(Second Interview, Alesha's Mum and Aunt, *Genetic Journeys* project)

From a medicalisation point of view this statement, implying that somehow Alesha was in the diagram, could be seen as an example of medicine's ability to provide the master narrative that objectifies the person; containing them within a medical framework that positions them as different. However, the mother's account of the diagram and its relationship to her daughter did not objectify and stigmatise her in the straightforward way medicalisation would imply. Instead her mum drew out a meaning for the diagram that was positive – the language she constantly returned to was of uniqueness – and relational to the other aspects of Alesha that were sustained in her life within the family. This echoed a comment a young girl from another family in the study made following being told by a geneticist that both her and her mother shared the same genetic variation. This variation, the geneticist believed, explained why both shared differences in their cognitive development. Alice, when asked by us what she felt about this, said it made her happy because it meant 'we are the same' (One-Off Interview, Alice, *Genetic Journeys* project). The medical narrative of difference was drawn in different ways in these two cases – in one to celebrate uniqueness, in the other to celebrate sameness – into kinship narratives that enabled them to be interpreted outside of stigma and objectification.

While the diagram was an artefact that could symbolise an aspect of a child's personhood as different from others, it was limited in defining the scope of that personhood now and into the future. Its limits came from two sources. First, it sits alongside other narratives that 'hold' a personhood together. One such narrative, but there are others, are the ties of kinship (Lindemann, 2014). As we shall explore in Chapter 6, kinship is not inherently positive in its link to person-hood, but here we see how it can be in providing non-stigmatising accounts of what makes a person who they are. The second reason is that the diagram offers one description of one aspect of who a child is. Alesha's mum in the same inter-view talked about how genetics was only one aspect of her child's life. Genetics had provided some form of explanation and now their focus was much more on looking after Alesha and aiding her to develop in ways that would not be a result of genetics, but of care. Alesha was not in the diagram, she was alive, in her home playing. While watching Alesha, with the diagram left to the side, her mum went on to say:

> What they've said at genetics is they can't say exactly how the chromosome disorder will affect her, because Alesha is unique. But at the moment, most days, I don't even think about it. I just concentrate on getting on with what she needs, and stimulating her as much as I can. [Pause] But then I do think about it – I remember I have a daughter with special needs, she's going to have a different life to what we'd planned.... Genetics have told me as much as they know. So it's a case of like it or lump it, and I just put it at the back of my mind and don't think about it. I have accepted it. And, at the end of the day, she will still have a good life – it will just be different to the one we had expected. But she will still be loved and able to do as much as she is able to.
>
> (Second Interview, Alesha's Mum and Aunt, *Genetic Journeys* project)

Once the diagram and text that visualises Alesha's genetic difference entered the relational spaces and connections of family it remained an artefact of display and meaning. However, this occurred through how it was incorporated into the broader versions of Alesha that were maintained by those around her. This wider network – one centred on care – was seeking to create a different version of childhood and the future that genetics was a part of, but was not the definer of.

Diagnostic processes aiming to establish why a child's development is dif-ferent generate understandings that emphasise difference and disorder. The con-temporary fascination with tracing down the precise nature of how our genes vary carries the risk of such variations being used to categorise children into dif-ferent types – regardless of whether they can be linked to any symptoms or prob-lems in development or illness. How those categories are then taken up by other institutions such as education and welfare, can also play into their ability to segregate disabled children and young people into different social positions and spaces. Linking difference in child development to differences in genetic make-up may be productive of broader institutional and societal monitoring dynamics that treat variation as problematic and something to be intervened in (including influencing the subsequent reproductive choices of the parent or into the future the child themselves). However, the full scope of what genetics, or any other diagnostic process brings, will not just be a product of medicine on its own. Broader 'relations of exchange' are vital to exploring how understandings produced via medical diagnosis become incorporated into ongoing sources of defining difference and disorder. Kinship, as will be explored in Chapter 6, is an important source of meaning and identity, as well as a site of scrutiny and monitoring of children. Our account of the diagnostic process has emphasised the work parents do to make sense of what medicine seeks to say about and do with their child. It is also important we look at what children and young people themselves think and do. To do that we turn to an exploration of medical intervention.

Medical intervention

What follows diagnosis is treatment and intervention (although not straight forwardly in the case of genetics as identification of genetic variation does not always generate treatment options). The form of treatment will vary but depending on the diagnosis it can be medication, speech or behavioural therapy, physiotherapy, the wearing of various medical supports such as splints or surgery. Such interventions have a variety of purpose, our interest here is with those that seek to minimise difference, approximate normality in areas such as movement and speech and aim to enable independence (Parens, 2006). For children and young people with mobility issues this can include multiple surgeries to straighten limbs, ensure they walk more normally and remain out of a wheelchair. Medication is increasingly used in the Global North as a way to contain the 'disturbance' children who have been diagnosed with conditions such as ADHD or autistic spectrum disorder are said to have on the operation and regulation of public space. Across these treatments the intent is that by 'normalising' disabled children their opportunities to progress in society and be independent will be improved. However, from a disability studies perspective this is a deeply suspect medical response to disability. First, it neglects the role of medicine in the production of understandings of difference as problematic in the first place. Second, parents who consent for such interventions to occur, while wishing the best for their child, are also in the process contributing to the social dis-valuing of the differences their children embody (Hansen and Hansen, 2006). Third, if the goal is to ensure a better fit between the child and social norms and structures, then it is a solution that appears to prioritise fixing the child, over fixing or challenging those existing and discriminatory social norms and structures. It is the child who should monitor their behaviour to conform as much as possible, who should have their senses dulled by pharmaceutical solutions and who should undertake painful and repeated surgeries to enable their bodies to appear as others would like them to look.

Children and young people themselves are important actors in the process as they must be actively involved; whether participating in physiotherapy, wearing medical devices such as splints, or managing the pain and discomfort that comes with surgery. In their early years it is parents and medical actors who play the major role in deciding what will be attempted, as children get older their perspective becomes increasingly important, both in terms of decisions they make about agreeing to intervention, but also through how they go about their participation in such interventions. Here we want to explore how disabled children and young people we have worked with engage with medical intervention, and how they situate it within their broader social worlds and aspirations for the future. Through doing so, again, medicine is placed within broader 'relations of exchange' that influence children and young people's approach to it.

In the *Embodied Transitions* project an area of particular focus was the past and current medical interventions the participants had experienced. A diagnosis of cerebral palsy at or around birth commonly leads to a cycle of intervention across childhood and into adolescence. A significant focus of such interventions – with surgery and long term physiotherapy at the centre – is to aid mobility, strength and dexterity. Such interventions are also supported by young people wearing technologies such as splints to train muscles and bones to move and grow in particular ways. Pharmaceuticals are often used as well, both managing pain and aiding muscles to work in controlled ways. This range of intervention has embedded within it a clear message that to walk is better than not to and that to walk as normally as possible is a good thing. This holds too for other aspects that can be affected by cerebral palsy such as speech and arm movement. The explicit aim is that in the present and in the future the child will be able to be more independent by being less reliant on assistive technology and others. Therefore, here we have the template example of the medical response to embodied difference being to work towards minimising that difference as much as possible. This template lies at the centre of disability studies' distrust of medicine. Its focus on fixing where possible, turns the different body into the disabled body (Davis, 1995).

We do not want to suggest disability studies is wrong to be critical of medicine and its response to childhood disability. However, we want to examine how medicine sits alongside other institutions and practices that valorise normality, and to consider how disabled children and young people themselves approach their interactions with it. A standard medicalisation approach might propose that disabled children and young people are embedded in cycles of intervention that they have undertaken since birth. A cycle which leads them to incorporate such practices without question. Understanding young people's relationship to medical imperatives in this way is risky. It treats young people as passive recipients incapable of questioning what is happening to them. Instead, as childhood studies reminds us, it is important to think about how young people, as 'experiencing agents' (Kelly, 2005), situate medical practices within their social worlds. Here we want to draw from the *Embodied Transitions* project to explore how young people who have grown up in a context of medical therapies trying to normalise their bodies respond as they enter adolescence. We are interested in how medical imperatives of fixing are drawn into the personhood the young people are shaping and enacting. Is medicalisation all that is happening in these cycles of repair and desires for normalcy? What broader social and personal narratives may also be present as informing 'choices' to participate in painful medical practices?

Medical bodies

During our first interviews with the young people in the project, the participants reflected on how medical interventions were important elements of their childhood. Many discussed, in matter of fact ways, multiple surgeries, regular physiotherapy, injections of muscle relaxant and the wearing of medical devices such as splints and callipers:

SARA: I had four I think, first one was putting plates in my knees, [pause] and putting cow bone into my foot.... The second one was putting wire into my foot, or taking the wire out, no taking the wire out it was. So I had wire put in my foot, and I had that taken out, and the third one was having my tendons stretched from my hip to my foot I think, so I've got, like, a big scar at the back of my leg, so that was quite sore, but yeah I got that over and done with. And then the fourth one was just taking the plates they put in the first time out.

INTERVIEWER: So why was it that they did all these things?

SARA: It's just to straighten my legs I think? 'Cos when I walk I have a bit of a crouch, so I think that's why they put it in just to sort of make me look a bit more normal, does that make sense?

(One-Off Interview, Sara, *Embodied Transitions* project)

Sara's account is typical of the level of intervention experienced in childhood. While there was acknowledgement of some of the costs of those interventions – time spent away from school, family and friends, periods of intense pain – there was little sense in the interviews they had done as children in the SPARCLE project, or in their interviews with us, that such interventions were themselves questioned or unusual. Instead, they presented these changes to their body as something they had, for the most part, benefited from:

I think I do have a good future.... Like what I would be able to do now after I've had me operations and that. And just like I'll definitely be able to be more independent, like if I didn't have the operations. So it's making a lot better.... With me walking and like growing up.

(Interview One, Paul, *Embodied Transitions* project)

These past interventions reshaped their bodies, and the way they spoke of them also narratively framed their bodies as in need of repair. Their accounts of improvement emphasised that the childhood body should be seen as an object of change, something that could/should be remade in the ways medicine made possible. Both Sara and Paul's quotes emphasise that embedded in the interventions was the goal of making the body function 'better', to both appear as normal as possible and enable independence. This objective remained in interventions that were carrying on into the present day. Hannah, for instance, spoke and represented her childhood surgeries quite negatively and indicated that she had withdrawn from more surgeries because of the pain involved and the disruption they created:

I've been in and out of hospitals, I've been poked and prodded and I think I just got fed up of being like poked and prodded and operated on and I think I just got sick of being in there getting things done.

(Interview One, Hannah, *Embodied Transitions* project)

Hannah also captured her negative association with childhood interventions in her journal, where in images such as Figure 4.1, she represented them via images of medical equipment, hospital beds and pain. However, in the same interview she explained that she had decided to have further surgery on her hand and leg. The aim was in part to alleviate pain, but also, as she said in her photo-elicitation interview after the surgery, to straighten her legs out; to make them more 'normal', something she reinforced by gesturing towards the body of the interviewer:

…now it's not completely straight, they can't get it like yours, they can't get it, it's too strong but basically now it's like that, like still turned in a bit but more straighter than before. They can't get it like a normal, basically I won't get a normal foot, but it's to me it's more normal than what it was if you know what I mean by that, but it doesn't look like say your foot, but to me it's normal because it's like kind of like other people's. Does that make sense?

(Interview Two, Hannah, *Embodied Transitions* project)

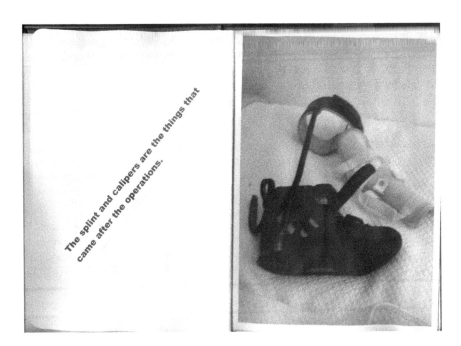

Figure 4.1 Journal, Hannah, *Embodied Transitions* project.

In Hannah's journal she put two pictures of her arm and leg bandaged and in plaster and wrote alongside 'pain surgery'.

Hannah associated the surgeries with pain, and captured that association powerfully in her journal (see Figures 4.2 and 4.3), yet in her interview spoke of her own choice to undertake the procedure. Her photographs, in part through how they separated out the part of the body being worked on by medicine, represents how intervention dissects the body in order that aspects of it become objects of intervention. Alongside, the interview bore testimony to the desire for normality as a contributor to a decision to participate in such painful surgery.

Hannah's account, across textual and visual representations, emphasises the medical reshaping of the material body that had begun in childhood but continued to the present day. She highlights how young people are drawn into a cycle of approaching the body as something to be worked on, even when they also acknowledged the effects of being 'poked at'. The medical imperative to fix, their familiarity with medical procedures, changes to the body that led to pain, produced a practice that opened up elements of the body to intervention, which stories of promised improvement in function and appearance supported. As Hoffman (2013) argues medical interventions tutor those receiving them into engaging with their bodies as something to work on. Even though surgery brought pain and disruption it was experienced as a commonplace activity to be returned to if the body slipped away from normality in its shape and function. Through this cycle of activity they were drawn into medicine's advocacy of

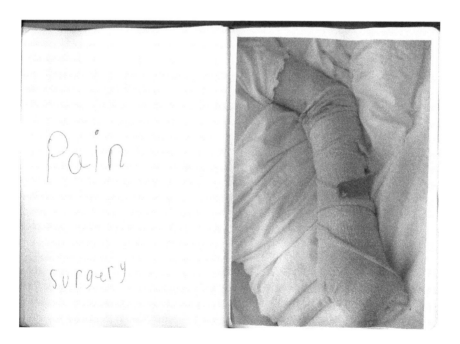

Figure 4.2 Journal, Hannah, *Embodied Transitions* project.

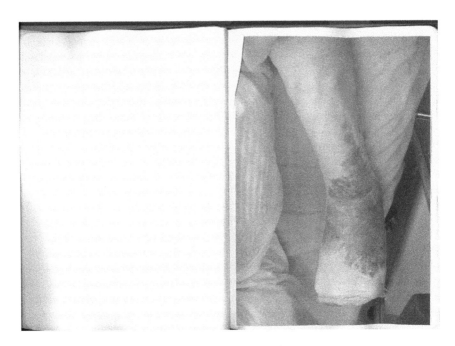

Figure 4.3 Journal, Hannah, *Embodied Transitions* project.

intervention; an advocacy that privileged doing things normally and being independent over other forms of embodiment and interaction with the world.

Disability and its medical management was, in this way, a continuous thread
in the young people's lives that had not lessened in significance as they got
older. The majority of the participants were still receiving regular physiotherapy,
often augmented by their own trips to the gym or swimming pool and regular
exercises at home:

INTERVIEWER: What kind of exercises are you doing, stretching?

ANDREW: Yeah just stretching doing this [stretching ankle], going on the bottom
stairs just dropping my heel that kind of thing, and just going to the wall and
just pushing against the wall and just getting this leg back and then stretching here [pats right hamstring].

(One-Off Interview, Andrew, *Embodied Transitions* project)

The prominence of this cycle in the young people's lives raises a number of
issues. The one we would like to highlight here is the relationship to the body it
created. While the young people spoke positively about how medicine and their
own activities such as exercise could enable them to be more normal, there was
also recognition that they would never quite reach normality. As the body grew
this could undermine the progress that had been made, triggering, as it had for
Hannah, a return to the operating table and the physiotherapist:

When I was five I used to be able to climb up the windows, but I can't do that now ... my muscles have got tighter and my body has got tighter. I wasn't in as much pain when I was young but now I am in a lot more pain ... I am growing; obviously my muscles aren't long enough because they stop at a certain amount. Basically, I've got the muscles of an eleven year old, instead of a fifteen year old, and I have to get a lot of surgery to make them long enough.

(One-Off Interview, Emma, *Embodied Transitions* project)

Their bodies were located between two poles – a 'normal' non-impaired body always to be worked towards, and the 'flawed' body of cerebral palsy. While they and medicine could work to improve their bodies; their relationship to their bodies was one which emphasised its capacity to let them – and medicine – down. This was evidenced in the way several participants framed cerebral palsy as possibly undermining the lives they were living and the futures they were making. For example, at different points Mark spoke about walking, initially speaking with pride about still being 'on his feet', and demonstrating photographically (see Figure 4.4) the work he does to stay that way. During his second interview however, he reflected on the transience of that, indicating how changes to the body would eventually lead him to the wheelchair:

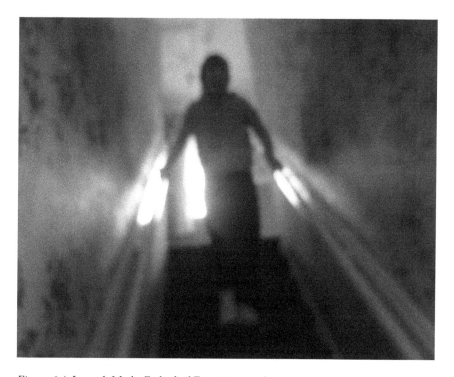

Figure 4.4 Journal, Mark, *Embodied Transitions* project.

> I think to get where I am with this disability is a good thing, I'd say it were a great thing. I don't think anyone that's got this far and still on their feet which uh, not being nasty, but not many people are on their feet with this disability. I very rarely see anyone on their feet with this disability ... I'm still on my feet at seventeen and with a bit of weight about me, it's pretty much a good thing.
>
> (Interview One, Mark, *Embodied Transitions* project)

> ... from what I've been looking at, when you get older, when you say you're fifty, well not when your middle-aged, I think you get, you'll be struggling to walk, because my joints are going, you know stuck in that position then, so your obviously, I'm never going to be able to walk properly and I'm never going to be able to walk from now until I pass away.
>
> (Interview Two, Mark, *Embodied Transitions* project)

The gap between medical promises of being able to remake their bodies as normal and the long term capacity of their bodies to fulfil that promise produced a mistrust of their bodies. Here we do see the potential harm embedded in medical practices that approach embodied differences as something to ideally be minimised, rather than lived with. It should not be forgotten that aspects of medical intervention can alleviate pain and enable greater participation in a society not designed for embodied difference; but nevertheless one cost is the unease it generates for the body unable to sustain medicine's goals.

Social bodies

In relation to genetic diagnosis we argued that medicine was not the only player in shaping its meaning and significance. This is also the case for thinking about both what relationship to the child/adolescent body medical interventions create and also why children and young people participate in them. Disabled children and young people are not just absorbing medical messages in their advocacy of intervention and normality. We need again to step out from medicine and look more broadly to the social value given to being normal and independent – as discussed in the previous chapter. The participants' own everyday comparisons with bodies they read as within the comfort and safety of normality encouraged both their own framing of their bodies as different and lesser and their pursuit of practices that could re-shape their body. This cycle of comparison and attempts towards normality were particularly notable amongst those with siblings who did not have a diagnosis of disability:

> I would just like to be treated as a person, just like how me brother's treated I would like to be treated in that way.
>
> ...
>
> Like when I went to college, I was the only one with a disability in the class, so when I started they were like 'Are you alright', or 'Can you go downstairs like that', I didn't like really like that.
>
> (Interview One, Paul, *Embodied Transitions* project)

Paul also discussed how in social spaces such as college he would adapt his movement and use of assistive technology in order to be interpreted by others as similar to them. When asked during his photo elicitation interview how he would like to be seen, Paul explained that he wanted to be recognised as 'ordinary'; this speaks to both the safety of normality and also the importance of the social context of adolescence and thoughts of adult futures to the relationship disabled young people have to their bodies.

It is not only the body that is changing as young people move through adolescence; teenage and adult identities and aspirations emerge too, and this temporal dimension also influenced how the young people thought about what they needed to do to keep their bodies functioning as well as possible. These aspirations and their desire to enact the socially recognisable forms of adult identity we highlighted in Chapter 3 were as important as any medical goals. Their own developing sense of self now and who they wanted to be in the future became vital to their approach to working on their body and their monitoring of it. Intervention changed in its meaning and focus. Whereas many young people spoke, as children, about impairment as a limitation on the extent to which they could play at their friends' houses or join in children's games. The older they got the more concerns turned to the ability to live much like other young men and women, including going out with friends, forming intimate and sexual relationships, being able to be self-reliant and living independently:

CRAIG: I use it [a hoist to get into the bath] more now, 'cos I'm getting older and I'm getting bigger. More preferable for me using that piece of equipment rather than my parents lifting me about so it's easier on the both sides.

INTERVIEWER: So do you think as you get older that being independent will get more important?

CRAIG: I'm a lot more independent now, compared to what I was then. Maybe if I get more independent things will be easier for me and for others. So it's better for me to be more independent. I'm going to be eighteen next year and I will need to be more independent. I'm going to want to go out drinking with mates, meeting girls. Not just these things but other things too, I'm going to want to live on my own someday. So I'm going to want to be more independent now, rather than waiting some years down the line.

(One-Off Interview, Craig, *Embodied Transitions* project)

Craig's version of who he wanted to be and the body that would enable him to be that person is filtered through gendered norms about what a young man's life should ordinarily include. Mark (as we mentioned in the last chapter) also spoke of how his hard fought mobility enabled him to stand at the bar drinking alcohol with his mates (although he needed to monitor how much he drank to ensure he did not fall over). The work they did via medical intervention and their own extensive work on their bodies were crafted from and drawn into their adolescent narratives about having an 'ordinary' body that could do 'ordinary' adolescent things:

SARA: I sort of try and steady myself, so I don't do too much and I don't do too little, because my problem is that I'm quite stubborn, so I don't tend to do too little anyway. I tend to just sort of do it all in one go … I just sort of go for it really.

INTERVIEWER: Why are you so insistent that you're going to do stuff?

SARA: Everything. Everything a normal person probably could do. But I have to sort of steady myself because obviously if I do too much then, say like my feet will hurt, or my ankles or whatever … I don't know like, the distance a person could walk, I tend to sort of think 'Oh no I'm fine', my mams like 'Do you want to sit down', and I'll be like 'no' [laughs].

(One-Off Interview, Sara, *Embodied Transitions* project)

The bodies medicine had sought to create during their childhood, against norms of body function and appearance, were now bodies they sought to create against norms that mattered to them, including keeping up with peers and living as 'capable' young men and women. Through their varied responses to seeking to match their bodies to their adolescent identities and their adult aspirations we can see their body symbolically and materially changing. Medical imperatives to fix and re-fix, join with social desires to do everyday ordinary things in ordinary ways, to provide a different rationale for the importance of always working on the body. Getting older, and being older, placed new expectations on the body, and on 'doing', which the young people sought to embody as they negotiated the transition into adulthood. These practices ran alongside the surgical transformations they were undertaking to normalize the body.

Several participants in the *Embodied Transitions* project gave the example of making a cup of tea by themselves. It was both something that could prove their ability to live independently through, but also something they worked very hard to build up their dexterity and strength in order to do. The micro-management and commitment involved in making a body that can do something as common place as make a cup of tea, shows the deep embedded nature of norms of independence as self-reliance in people's understandings of who is the valued subject.

What such attempts to do normal things normally also emphasise is that normal embodiment is something that involves placing disability into the background by re-training the body to do things the way others do. Kate was keen to become a medical doctor, in preparation for that, and to prove to others it might be possible even with a body that was different, she had spent hours training herself to be able to suture like an able-bodied person. She reflected on both her ability to do the sutures and as above to make a cup of tea as proof of her similarity to others:

there is a set of things that you have to be able to do to become a doctor, but my GP is also a good friend of mine so he's taken me through each one of those things so the first one is suturing and the first few you know while I got used to it were not great but then the last few I got it off to a T and I could do it. It is just all about perseverance and that kind of thing so I mean by no means are they hugely effective it's just things like if I was writing a long piece of writing in class my hand would get tired and so then someone would have to come and scribe for me or things like pouring occasionally pouring something from one container into another is difficult but if I really do concentrate I can do it like I can make cups of tea and stuff so I can pour the kettle in to the cup so it's just it's just very, very little effect really.

(Interview One, Kate, *Embodied Transitions* project)

The body thus becomes a tool in the enactment of not just independence but in proving a version of self-worth that is tied to achievement and self-realisation:

And in that way it's still the same with able bodied people because all they'll ever do is do stuff to the best of their ability so then not that you weren't originally but from the outside world you can do stuff to the same level.

(Interview One, Kate, *Embodied Transitions* project)

The influence of the identity work of the young people complicates the medicalisation account in two important ways. First, medicine is not alone in the valorisation of normality and independence. The social valuing of such norms as symbolic of successful transitions to adulthood are crucial in young people's compliance with medical procedures. The medical and social work together to validate the norms young people aspire to. Second, there is clearly the kinds of self-disciplining and self-monitoring present here that is associated with medicalisation. The young people measured themselves against other body norms and worked towards what and who they wanted to be. However, there are productive forms of agency also present in the pleasure they took in remaking their bodies, in imagining adult futures, and in their participation in choices about whether to have another surgery, in whether to swim another lap. They did not passively go along with what medicine said, instead they were embedded in ongoing processes of forming and doing their relational identity through their situated pursuit of everyday ordinariness as normality.

Conclusion

Medicine remains a central institution that promotes the value of normality and closely associates having a body that can enact independence as central to that normality. Its practices of diagnosis aid delineations between normal and abnormal bodies and its multiple modes of intervention act upon those placed in the category of abnormality. However, this does not capture all that is happening in the interaction between those bodies it diagnoses and intervenes upon. Other practices, other discourses and narratives from broader social and cultural landscapes are involved in mediating medicine's influence. Some of those broader landscapes or social worlds, such as family and kinship, hold the disabled child or young person within the category of normality; others, such as the social value placed on normality and independence, emphasise the work the disabled child or young person must first undertake in order to be recognised by others as normal.

References

Asberg, C. and Johnson, E. (2009) Viagra selfhood: pharmaceutical advertising and the visual formation of Swedish masculinity. *Health Care Analysis*, 17(2): 144–157.

Asberg, C. and Lum, J. (2009) Pharmad-ventures: a feminist analysis of the pharmaco-logical imaginary of Alzheimer's disease. *Body & Society*, 15(4): 95–117.

Barnes, C. and Mercer, G. (2010) *Exploring Disability*. Cambridge: Polity Press.

Baudrillard, J. (1994) *Simulacra and Simulation*. Ann Arbor, MI: University of Michigan Press.

Birke, L. (1999) *Feminism and the Biological Body*. Edinburgh: Edinburgh University Press.

Bleakley, A. and Bligh, J. (2009) Who can resist Foucault? *Journal of Medicine and Philosophy*, 34(4): 368–383.

Braidotti, R. (2002) *Metamorphoses: Towards a Materialist Theory of Becoming*. Cambridge: Polity Press.

Buchbinder, M. and Timmermans, S. (2011) Medical technologies and the dream of the perfect newborn. *Medical Anthropology*, 30(1): 56–80.

Clarke, A.E. and Fujimura, J.H. (eds) (1992) *The Right Tools for the Job: At Work in the Twentieth Century Life Sciences*. Princeton, NJ: Princeton University Press.

Conrad, P. (1992) Medicalization and social control. *Annual Review of Sociology*, 18: 209–232.

Conrad, P. and Schneider, J.W. (1980) *Deviance and Medicalization: From Badness to Sickness*. St Louis, MS: C.V. Mosby.

Davis, L.J. (1995) *Enforcing Normalcy: Disability, Deafness and the Body*. London: Verso.

Draper, J. (2002) 'It was a really good show': the ultrasound scan, fathers and the power of visual knowledge. *Sociology of Health & Illness*, 24(6): 771–795.

Edwards, J. (2005) 'Make-up': personhood through the lens of biotechnology. *Ethnos*, 70(3): 413–431.

Featherstone, K., Atkinson, P., Bharadwaj, A. and Clarke, A. (2006) *Risky Relations: Family Kinship and the New Genetics*. Oxford: Berg.

Featherstone, K., Latimer, J., Atkinson, P., Pilz, D.T. and Clarke, A. (2005) Dysmorphol-ogy and the spectacle of the clinic. *Sociology of Health & Illness*, 27(5): 551–574.

Feder, E.K. (2008) Imperatives of normality: from 'intersex' to 'disorders of sex develop-ment'. *GLQ*, 15(2): 225–247.

Foucault, M. (1975) *The Birth of the Clinic*. New York, NY: Vintage Books.

Foucault, M. ([1976] 1990) *The History of Sexuality, Vol. 1: An Introduction*. London: Penguin Books.

Hansen, D.L. and Hansen, E.H. (2006) Caught in a balancing act: parents' dilemmas regarding their ADHD child's treatment with stimulant medication. *Qualitative Health Research*, 16(9): 1267–1285.

Haraway, D.J. (1991) *Simians, Cyborgs and Women: The Reinvention of Nature*. New York, NY: Routledge.

Hoffman, M. (2013) Bodies completed: on the physical rehabilitation of lower limb amputees. *Health*, 17(3): 229–245.

Illich, I. (1976) *Medical Nemesis: The Expropriation of Health*. New York, NY: Pantheon.

Kelly, S.E. (2005) 'A different light' – examining, impairment through parent narratives of childhood disability. *Journal of Contemporary Ethnography*, 34(2): 180–205.

Latimer, J. (2013) *The Gene, the Clinic and the Family*. London: Routledge.

Ledbetter, D.H. (2008) Cytogenetic technology – genotype and phenotype. *New England Journal of Medicine*, 359(16): 1728–1730.

Lindemann, H. (2014) *Holding and Letting Go*. Oxford: Oxford University Press.

McLaughlin, J. and Clavering, E.K. (2012) Visualising difference, similarity and belonging in paediatric genetics. *Sociology of Health and Illness*, 34(3): 459–474.

Mol, A. (2002) *The Body Multiple: Ontology in Medical Practice*. Durham, NC: Duke University Press.

Navon, D. (2011) Genomic designation: how genetics can delineate new, phenotypically diffuse medical categories. *Social Studies of Science*, 41(2): 203–226.

Newman, J. and Vidler, E. (2006) Discriminating customers, responsible patients, empowered users: consumerism and the modernisation of health care. *Journal of Social Policy*, 35(2): 193–209.

Nishizaka, A. (2011) The embodied organization of a real-time fetus: the visible and invisible in prenatal ultrasound examinations. *Social Studies of Science*, 41(3): 309–336.

Novas, C. and Rose, N. (2000) Genetic risk and the birth of the somatic individual. *Economy and Society*, 29(4): 485–513.

Parens, E. (ed.) (2006) *Surgically Shaping Children: Technology, Ethics and the Pursuit of Normality*. Baltimore, MD: The Johns Hopkins University Press.

Petchesky, R.P. (1987) Foetal images: the power of visual culture in the politics of reproduction. *Feminist Studies*, 13(2): 263–292.

Roberts, J. (2012) 'Wakey wakey baby': narrating four-dimensional (4D) bonding scans. *Sociology of Health & Illness*, 34(2): 299–314.

Rose, N. and Novas, C. (2005) Biological citizenship. In A. Ong, and S.J. Collier (eds), *Global Assemblages: Technology, Politics, and Ethics as Anthropological Problems*. pp. 439–463. Oxford: Blackwell.

Shildrick, M. (2005) The disabled body, genealogy and undecidability. *Cultural Studies*, 19(6): 755–770.

Stiker, H.-J. (2000) *A History of Disability*. Ann Arbor, MI: The University of Michigan Press.

Strathern, M. (1992) *After Nature: English Kinship in the Late Twentieth Century*. Cambridge: Cambridge University Press.

Wilson, E.A. (2004) *Psychosomatic: Feminism and the Neurological Body*. Durham, NC: Duke University Press.

Zechmeister, I. (2001) Foetal images: the power of visual technology in antenatal care and the implications for women's reproductive freedom. *Health Care Analysis*, 9: 387–400.

Part III
Relational identity and practice

5 Embodied practices and valued identities

In the previous two chapters we focused on institutions of childhood. We showed how relational dynamics around interactions, and the enactment of identity, influenced the presence of institutions in disabled children and young people's lives. How institutions impart values of normality and produce disability categories is mediated by the ways in which people interact within them, drawing into those interactions other players in the production of norms and otherness. In this chapter, and the next, we flip the focus round to exploring the relationship between different aspects of identity and embodiment, which occur in different sites across the social world and through which disabled children and young people play key roles in shaping the significance of those interactions and what that means for their identity. In this chapter we focus on embodiment, in particular the range of embodied practices disabled children and young people participate in. The following chapter explores the disruption and maintenance of belonging within families that can occur in contexts of childhood disability.

Disability studies is known for its disquiet with analyses of the body (Williams, 1999). Its concern is that a focus on the body takes us back into medical understandings of personal tragedy and an individualised approach to impairment (Barnes, 2012). However, for some time this exclusion has been queried from within disability studies (Marks, 1999; Paterson and Hughes, 1999; Snyder and Mitchell, 2001; Wendell, 1996). As indicated in Chapter 1, this has led to an expansive period of work on disability that takes seriously the social significance of how we think about and live in our bodies. The research that has emerged on embodied disability rejects the argument that a concern with bodies leads to an emphasis on tragedy. Instead, the work is interested in 'people's innovative strategies to negotiate living with(in) their bodies in their everyday social lives' (Zitzelsberger, 2005: 350), as well as exploring how the body sits 'at the intersection of culture, society, and embodiment' (Hammer, 2012: 410). The approach is focused on, first, the aspects of our lives that, while influenced by material relations, are not determined by them, and second, the dimensions of marginality and discrimination that generate losses that are not just economic and political (Thomas, 2002). By doing so, it allows for investigations into the relationship between claims to normality and the dynamics of monitoring, regulation and resistance. As Garland-Thomson argues (2007: 114), cultural stories about the normal or the 'normate' 'structure our shapes' through the interrelationship between the stories we tell and the things we do to, and with, our bodies in response to the versions of normality that appear important to us and others.

We draw such approaches into a consideration of disabled childhoods because the scrutiny that falls on disabled children and young people's different bodies is not just a formal dynamic of structures of categorisation and rules of appropriateness. It is also the everyday scrutiny that occurs between social actors as they negotiate their way in the world; making discourse into practice and enacting identities that self-discipline and -regulate, and resist and recreate. This chapter will explore how an interest in disabled embodiment can be a fruitful way to 'flesh out' how disabled children and young people are monitored, regulated and marginalised, and their responses to such practices and positionings. After laying out some of the particular theoretical tools we are using to engage with relational embodiment, we will explore how children and young people across our projects were involved in a series of ongoing 'body projects'. We will make a distinction between projects that positioned disability in the background as they strove for the sanctuary of adolescent ordinariness, and others that enacted a valued identity through, rather than despite, their different embodiments.

Working on the body

In Chapter 1 we explored the overlap and distinction between the ways in which we engage with embodiment and how critical disability studies does. Before exploring the embodied practices of the disabled children and young people we have worked with, we wish to explain our approach to embodied practice and its relationship to discourse through going back to that discussion.

Critical disability studies proposes that the turning of difference into disability (and impairment) is a result of psychic and social discomfort with bodies that appear outside of the norms of a world that prides itself in its ability to progress and to conquer illness and fragility:

> In signifying disease, trauma and decay, the anomalous body is an uncomfortable reminder that the normative, 'healthy', body, despite its appearance of successful self-determination, is highly vulnerable to disruption and disease.
>
> (Shildrick, 2005: 757)

The possibility that bodies are forms of 'always already unstable corpus' (Shildrick, 1999: 77) is hidden behind modernist fantasises, encouraged by medicine, that imperfection can be remedied and that bodies should be able to enact autonomy. Bodies that appear not to work quite right highlight that all bodies matter and that minds are embedded in bodies that can fail. As Garland-Thomson (2007: 114) also argues, disabled people disclose 'the myth of certainty and compliancy in regard to human bodies'. Individual unease about the vulnerability of our own bodies, supported by cultural symbolism that also expresses such unease, encourages people to position certain ways of living and being as outside the possibilities of normalcy and humanness. Shildrick's account positions materiality as meaningful through discursive articulation. Without a discursive framing the normal could not be recognised; without bodies that cannot fit within that discursive framing, the normal could not be celebrated. This is an explicitly relational understanding of the body, which sees the juxtaposition of the normal alongside the abnormal as co-producing each other: 'The monstrous body, then, plays a key role in the construction and reinforcement of distinctions between normal and abnormal, and in the imposition of normativities' (Shildrick, 2005: 762). In critical disability studies the monstrous body (Braidotti, 1996) is thus defined as 'neither a biological nor sociological category, but an interface, a threshold, a field of intersecting material and symbolic forces; a surface where multiple codes (sex, class, age, race, etc.) are inscribed' (Goodley and Runswick-Cole, 2013: 5).

There is much we agree with in the priorities and concerns summarised above: the significance of language to the attribution of meaning to the body; the relational quality of such meanings; the importance of framing of the other or the abnormal, to enabling the 'normal' to be secured, celebrated and made real. However, we want to both work with and against these arguments in order to make a case for seeing the body as something more than an inert substance made 'real' (or of consequence) by language and psychic anxiety. In doing so we draw from writers within contemporary body studies who argue that '*Language has been granted* too much power' (original emphasis, Barad, 2003: 801). Such work is wary of the path Shildrick (2005) or Butler (1993) take us on, where the body itself appears to matter less than words or psychic processes. Rather like Thomas (2007) or Hughes (2009), we want to retain an interest in the material aspects of the body, without retreating back to a social model version of materiality:

> ...while impairment is not the cause of disability, it is the raw material upon which disability works. It is the embodied socio-biological substance – socially marked as unacceptable bodily deviation – that mediates the social relationships in question.
>
> (Thomas, 2004: 25)

We do so by acknowledging the relational quality of embodiment highlighted by Shildrick (1999), but add to this the argument that the material qualities of the body and the things it co-exists with matter to the relational networks that form around and through it. The body is *both* material and social:

> Bodies matter, both as socially biological organisms – as experiencing and acting masses of organs, flesh, bones, blood, and nerves – and as complex networks of signs that are read and used by their owners to communicate messages within particular settings.
>
> (Staples, 2011: 546)

Contemporary body studies retain a concern with culture, language and relationality, but add to it the assertion that materiality also has a role, which is more than the canvas on which those things play out (Mol, 2002). Feminist materialists such as Hennessy (1993) are important precursors through the ways in which they responded to the 'cultural turn' produced by postmodernism by advocating for approaches that acknowledge that culture cannot or should not be divorced from a range of material factors that are productive to its emergence, maintenance and ability to be significant to othering. The body is brought actively into relational accounts by proposing that its material aspects play a non-determining role in how those relations emerge and develop. These are ongoing processes of becoming, which place the emphasis on doings and practices: '*matter comes to matter* through the iterative interactivity of the world and its becoming' (original emphasis, Barad, 2003: 823). Discourse and material are therefore in a relationship of 'mutual entailment' within which how they interact in social worlds is given greater emphasis than linguistic delineation: 'If an object is real this is because it is part of a practice. It is reality *enacted*' (original emphasis, Mol, 2002: 44). Linguistic expression and psychic anxiety must be enacted to have significance and that enactment is done by bodies interacting with each other and other things – as well as language. Those interactions also then change the qualities of the linguistic expressions and psychic anxiety they enact. This framing escapes assuming an interest in materiality or the body is about placing limits on what is discursively possible, while drawing the social far more into our understandings of how bodies come to matter in particular ways. As Colls (2007: 354) proposes, this 'approach acknowledges the 'dynamism' of bodily matter or the capacities of matter to be implicated in the process of its own materialisation, and is therefore utilised as a way to challenge an understanding of matter as passive and inert'. Colls uses this approach to examine the production and policing of 'fat' bodies in order to highlight how fat is more than a representation of a body shape, but also a doing of a body shape. In particular, she argues women who explore their fat bodies as producing an excess which is pleasurable, noncontainable, active, and valuable indicate that it is possible through the unusual body to not just portray it as non-other, but to become non-other. As Colls implies here, this acknowledgement of what people do with their bodies, as well as the representational framings they must negotiate, is open to the ways in which such practices can provide points of resistance to those framings.

A number of accounts now exist using this kind of relational material understanding for thinking about how bodies that differ from norms of function and capacity are produced within the relationships they are part of. Hammer, who undertook interviews with Israeli visually impaired women, argues they draw on their bodies to 'control the other's gaze, and to be perceived *not only* as blind/disabled but *also* as a person who can display femininity and human subjectivity as well as claim a public social legitimacy' (original emphasis, Hammer, 2012: 418). Staples (2011: 548) explores how specific material conditions in India 'literally create differently impaired bodies' and influence the ways in which such specific body differences are 'socially manifest' in the 'combined performances of a complex mesh of social agents'. Likewise, Hoffman (2013) links body techniques of rehabilitation favoured by medicine in Israel to the state validation of the heroic able-bodied military citizen, or what others have referred to as 'Israeli ableism' (Hammer, 2012; Mor, 2006).

Thinking about the relational production of bodies is particularly useful when researching children (Brownlie and Sheach Leith, 2011; Gottlieb, 2004; Lee and Motzkau, 2011; Mayall, 1996). It enables us to follow through with the childhood studies call to bring children and young people's situated agency into our examination, without falling into some important analytical and political traps. First, it does not understand agency as an individual property; instead it is emergent in the relations between children and young people and the things and people around them, which in practice afford certain avenues for influencing identity and social position (Kirk, 2010; Söderström, 2009). Second, as well as being acutely open to such agency dynamics, it also remains aware of the regulatory dynamics that influence the operation of localised relational embodied networks, as available social norms and values pervade actors' passage through the world and everyday opportunities for recognition and misrecognition. Finally, it is not forgetful of material inequalities that provide differential access to a range of actual resources and, more broadly, capital, which help secure existing social norms and values.

In what follows, we will detail the varied ways disabled children and young people in our projects have pursued a range of embodied work, influenced by multiple social norms and interactions, mediated by technology and productive of their emerging identities and patterns of inclusion and exclusion.

Social interaction and space

A focus on interactions leads to a consideration of how social space is a significant arena for the othering of those whose bodies appear to differ from norms of appearance and function (Freund, 1988, 2001; Kitchin, 1998). It is not just that such interactions occur within social spaces, but that the composition of space itself plays a part in the relational networks that monitor and produce notions of normality and difference around and through bodies (Imrie, 2001, 2013). Garland-Thomson suggests that one of the key forms of interaction that occurs between those who see themselves as within the boundaries of normate embodiment and those who are seen as outside is staring – an embodied practice, which may include linguistic exchange, but cannot be narrowed to that. Staring, Garland-Thomson argues, turns 'the disabled subject into a grotesque spectacle, the stare is the gesture that creates disability as an oppressive social relationship' (1997: 26) and positions some as removed from humanity: 'We may gaze at what we desire, but we stare at what astonishes us' (Garland-Thomson, 2006: 174). Associated with staring are a range of social practices – being laughed at, name called and ridiculed – that highlight: 'To be perceived as differently embodied … is still to occupy a place defined as exceptional, rather than to simply be part of a multiplicity of possibilities' (Shildrick, 2012: 31).

Practices of staring, ridicule and explicit hostility were common experiences narrated to us by children, young people and their families (as other researchers have found (Goodley and Runswick-Cole, 2011)):

> I find, like, if I just walk sometimes people will just stare and it really irritates us sometimes.... I don't know, it's just with, like, when I go for me dinner I'll go into [city] town centre and they kind of like, people that don't know you, haven't seen before and they just like have a little glare at you. I just think it's kind of rude, kind of just irritates me sometimes.
>
> (Interview One, Paul, *Embodied Transitions* project)

Paul's body became socially different through the ways in which the practice of staring marked it as worthy of a particular way of looking at it. The prevalence of the stare is supported by a social norm that says it is OK to find different embodiment unusual and to make your assessment known. Therefore the spaces in which bodies exist and the interactions they inform are important elements of the relational quality of body differences, as well as being productive to different forms of self-monitoring and social control. Emily, in the *Genetic Journeys* project, was unusually short against markers of normal child development. Having at a younger age been given hormone injections to try to increase her height, as she entered adolescence she went back to endocrinology to consider doing so once again. Her interest in using hormones to encourage height growth was explicitly linked to the fact that she was due to begin secondary school and her height difference would be more marked in that space. Emily also disliked that mothers at the school gate regularly picked her up and commented on how cute she looked. Something, as with other social reactions to body difference, she felt infantilised her. Her own monitoring of her body difference was encouraged by the social monitoring around her and led her to consider the kinds of medical fixing we discussed in the last chapter (Parens, 2006). Connor's mother in the *Genetic Journeys* project also discussed whether her young son should take hormones to help his growth. Both son and mother were significantly shorter than average height, the mother acknowledged difficulties she had faced due to her shortness (often being thought of as significantly younger than she was and assumed to have difficulties coping as an adult), however she felt that Connor was likely to suffer more due to his height because of his gender:

> ...like it's alright for now, but I don't think he'll be, 'cos they're saying that he's going to be smaller than me, and I'm only four foot eleven. And I don't think that, I don't really want him to be smaller than me, when he's a fully grown adult. I think it would stop him from doing a lot of stuff and would be like low in self-confidence and stuff. 'Cos I didn't like being this little, and I'm a girl, which I think it would be even more an issue if you were a boy.
>
> (One-Off Interview, Connor's Mum, *Genetic Journeys* project)

Social norms that associate appropriate masculinity with, at the very least, average height, gave greater emphasis to Connor's smallness being problematic and therefore something to be managed and fixed if at all possible.

In contrast, Liam, also from the *Genetic Journeys* project, was unusually tall for his age, something that was becoming more socially noticeable as his height increasingly became out of sync with his biological age. People expected him to be more 'mature' in his behaviour when they assumed he was older than he was, due to his body size. His school was struggling to incorporate him into the classroom space due to a lack of fit between his body and that environment: in particular they seemed unable to figure out what to do about his body being too big for the tables used for his year group:

> The occupational therapist has actually raised an issue. She said she had to go back into school in July to check Liam out. And I kind of thought you know, why? 'Because, you know, there was a really huge issue.' I said well what's the problem? She said, 'tables.' Sorry? 'Size of the tables, he just fits under them now and the tables don't get any bigger when he's in year three.' I went, right, okay, [laughs] I said so get a bigger table, and I said, or we've collected some beer mats for you if you want [laughs]. Again, I thought *that* is the problem, the tables!
>
> (Interview Two, Liam's Mum, *Genetic Journeys* project)

The mismatch between Liam's body and the material objects that fill the space he exists within at school, alongside the lack of creativity within the school on how to respond to that mismatch, together position Liam as out of place in his school and different from the others found there.

A bigger table will enable Liam to sit in his classroom, but there is also a risk that the different artefact, alongside his different body, will also become an element of the spatial relationships marking him as different to his classmates. The artefacts and technologies, which are part of many disabled children's lives, can encourage those around them in school, in the family and wider community to position them as different (Fenton *et al.*, 2013). This is not an inherent quality of the technology, but is produced through the interactions that form through them and the discursive framings available to explain them. Each play a part. Malik, from the *Embodied Transitions* project, used a communication device and spoke of the problems created by how people engage with those who use devices such as these (whose categorisation as assistive technology encourages the labelling of them and those that use them as different):

INTERVIEWER: What is bad about it?

MALIK: The public – people don't listen to wheelchair users, that's why it's difficult to talk to them.

INTERVIEWER: And do you ever find they don't listen to you?

MALIK: [Yeah]

INTERVIEWER: What do you think about that?

MALIK: I think it's bad because communication aid users, it takes a long time to talk.

INTERVIEWER: Do you find that people don't wait long enough for you to say something?

MALIK: Yes, that is what I am trying to say there.

INTERVIEWER: Why do you think that is?

MALIK: I don't know, but I think they should wait there.

(One-Off Interview, Malik, *Embodied Transitions* project)

Therefore an aid which may help keep someone alive, or aid mobility or communication, becomes a visible marker of difference through the ways in which people interact with the technology and the person connected to it:

> But now obviously she's got a tube in her stomach so they're now not sure of that, because the pump's still there. So the machinery's still around. So ... they're still thinking, 'oh she's still a sickly baby', and they just lobbed her into that again, the pigeon hole of, right she's got the medical problem, she's sick. So they won't actually come in and look after her. I mean, they're all concerned about her and they all ring up, and I mean they'll pop in every now and again but even that's gone down since, as she's getting older. Because obviously she's not at that little baby cutie stage anymore, so it's not where you can come and just have a cuddle, it's now she's more active so you've got to get down on your hands and knees and play and they're not sure about what they'll even do with her.
>
> (Interview One, Lauren's Mum, *Enabling Care* project)

Lauren's feeding tube was read as a visible reminder of her status as a medical object to be feared. The longer it stayed as she grew into a young child, the more it influenced the ways in which people continued to remain distant from her, emphasising in their enacted withdrawal that she was not quite 'one of us'.

Across these different social interactions, discomfort with difference, materialised via comparisons between different types of body and the reliance of some on medical or assistive technologies, leads to an awareness on the part of the children and young people and those around them that others are not quite sure how to engage with them, how to enable them to be participants in society. One response to this is to minimise these material symbols to difference in order to pass unnoticed through social space.

Background and ordinary

The everyday experiences of being stared at, which the young people had experienced all of their lives, led some to express a wish to be in the background and less noticeable. This was a practice that required that the markers of body difference should in some form be disguised or erased. Paul, who as we saw in the last chapter was keen to be seen as the same as other people, minimised his use of technologies that could help his mobility. When asked why he explained:

> Well I just don't, in a way I would like to take it with us. It is because a lot of people there are more likely just to stare 'cos I've got a stick. Just think it'll be easier to just not, without a stick.
>
> (Interview One, Paul, *Embodied Transitions* project)

The 'choice' to try to get about without a stick framed as an assistive technology that only people who are different use, echoes the refusal some expressed in Chapter 3 about receiving visible support from others. Because the technology and the act of support by another are both understood as only things certain kinds of bodies require, their presence provides a marker of difference as abnormality. This framing leads to a hesitance over using certain kinds of technology, which in itself leads to different embodied social practices. Someone like Paul then moves through social space without a walking stick or others avoid the use of a wheelchair if possible, because their use confirms to others they are different.

Desires to be less recognisable as different led also to body practices that aimed to disguise or hide markers of difference:

> When I was at school I always used to, 'cos we used to wear like long sleeves and that. And always did used to hide my hand and that, so people wouldn't see.
>
> (Interview One, Rachel, *Embodied Transitions* project)

In some cases this self-consciousness of how their bodies differed increased with adolescence – a period marked by hyper body surveillance and judgement (Guntram, 2013; Hauge and Haavind, 2011). When this occurred they became uncomfortable with social interactions that made their body differences visible to others, which previously they would have participated in.

> …in year seven to about year nine I used to wear shorts, I wasn't really bothered. I played basketball, I used to sit in the middle of the court and I used to be on both teams so if one team passed me the ball I'd pass it back to them and then if the other team wants it I passed it back to them, I was in the middle so I was like the playmaker, it was really good. When you were in like year seven and nine you don't really, well it didn't really matter what people thought of me and then when you got to year ten, eleven it was, I wanna wear trousers and not really be interested in PE if I'm gonna be sat in the middle looking like a fool, you know, er but it was good I enjoyed it but er looking back on it now it was a bit, sat in there everyone's running about and there's me sat in the middle of the court yeah…. I just think you start to wonder what people are gonna think of you. I used to wear shorts like I was saying for PE and now when in year ten I used to go in tracksuit bottoms

and, and I'm not letting anyone, don't like my legs, don't want people looking at my legs so I'd like cover them up.

(Interview One, Mark, *Embodied Transitions* project)

Mark, as part of his consciousness that his legs unsettled his integration into social relationships and spaces, also spoke of his desire to wear the same kind of stylish trainers that other young men wore, rather than the splints and supportive footwear he was supposed to wear to help his mobility and balance:

I was obviously going to stand out and say if you don't know me because I had sticks ... but like to have the Adidas, Nike or the Lacoste trainers that everyone else, my little way to sort of blend, you could sink into the background, not sink in the background, you wouldn't stand out, you know unless obviously you would but, I would like the Lacoste and Nike trainers, I don't know, buy the trainers you want, you'd sort of fit in a lot more.

(Interview Two, Mark, *Embodied Transitions* project)

While work on adolescent consumption tends to link the purchase of brand trainers with attempts to display individuality and fashionableness (Buckingham and Tingstad, 2010), for Mark, the focus was on achieving invisibility via the recognisability of such brands that other 'normal' people wore. Wearing such regular symbols of adolescent male fashion sense was thought of as a key through which entry to everyday culture could be obtained.

Attempts to move into the background encourage close surveillance and monitoring of intricate aspects of body movement, particularly if that movement was considered to be particularly odd or outside norms of how we are supposed to express our embodiment in the social world:

Because he's started developing some, almost like nervous ticks, which he's quite aware of now and he's becoming aware of some of his mannerisms and behaviours, and he's trying desperately to control them, in terms of the eye blinking. And the teacher has actually pulled me, and she thought he was asleep with his eyes wide open for about half an hour one afternoon. I said, no, it's because what he's realised is, that he's blinking too frequently. So what he'll try and do is actually control the blinking by keeping the eyes [widens eyes] to control the muscles to stop himself from doing it. Because he knows it's something which is odd and not right.

(Interview Three, Liam's Mother, *Genetic Journeys* project)

Liam's recognition that his body was developing in ways that seem different leads him to self-discipline, enacted through attempts to stop blinking – a response which itself generates other social questioning of his behaviour. In some ways he is in an unwinnable situation where norms of behaviour produce cycles of embodied monitoring of self and other that saturate his social space. Parents in our research could at times encourage their children to engage with this kind of self-monitoring, believing that ensuring their children fitted in better was an important task for them:

> But I really think it's made him a better person for it, he's a lot more normal if you like. We were trying to discourage him doing like the flapping hands and the pointed fingers and that. And if he gets really loud we'll say 'you know Jack you're shouting too loud and turn it down a bit'. He does take note of things like that I think because he wants to fit in, and I genuinely think he does want to fit in with other kids and what they're doing.
>
> (Interview Three, Jack's Mum, *Enabling Care* project)

Such monitoring practices signalled an attempt to be allowed into the category of the ordinary. Passing as ordinary, as in some way of little consequence, provides shelter from interactions that frame the person as extraordinary. The problem is that when ordinariness is sought through framing disability as absent or irrelevant, the social norm that difference is extraordinary remains unquestioned.

The quest, by parents, carers or young people to be recognised as socially valid subjects by minimising difference is understandable due to the penalties they experience in their social positioning as outside the norm. The consequences are important to consider in terms of rights and marginalisation and will be explored more fully in Chapter 7.

Refusing to pass

It would be wrong to suggest that seeking to pass and place disability into the background was the only response found amongst young people or their families. In a variety of ways, young people also sought to embody valued social positions that encompassed their different embodiment. However, in exploring encounters where difference was present it is important to distinguish between those where difference is 'allowed' or 'tolerated' and those where it does not ask for permission to be visible.

When difference is allowed its presence does not equate to an act of resistance and is instead contingent and contestable; this is because that presence still relies on others giving permission. Rachel, who as acknowledged earlier had hidden her hand in early secondary school, had stopped doing so when she realised others now accepted her body difference:

> Normally I think if people look at me and they think, you know, well she's got a disability, it doesn't matter as long as people see me for who I am and not somebody else. I'd rather somebody see me, having a disability but being able to get on with things and not looking as though it's effecting us really badly, it doesn't really matter how people see me. I mean obviously when I was younger people would look at us I would always, would think, what are they thinking, what they gonna think of what I look like, but as

I've grown older and more mature I've just learnt to take it on the chin and, you know, it doesn't matter if somebody looks at you a bit, you know, they might not be looking at you as to say oh she's got a disability, you know, she can't do this and that or.

(Interview Two, Rachel, *Embodied Transitions* project)

Rachel had developed greater scope to be in varied social spaces without hiding her embodied difference. However, at the same time it mattered to her that other people read that difference as insignificant to who she was. This need for others to see how she worked to make disability irrelevant meant that the social norms of overcoming disability remained the terms for entry. To some degree disability was now able to be displayed, but within ways that left existing social norms untroubled.

Disabled young people can, however, go further in challenging the monitoring power of understandings of normal bodies – here we will give three examples that do not require or indeed seek the permission of others. The first involves challenging those that seek to question their right to be within public space and to act in ways considered different from the norm:

...these lads laughed at me, 'cos I fell over and said something horrible and I will not repeat it, about my disability and one of my mates heard what they said, and my mate went 'What did you just say to my mate' and I had to grab hold of my mate and go 'No you don't' and pull them in the opposite direction. She said, 'We better leave, otherwise I am going to thump hhh. I went, 'No we're not going to punch people, we're going this way away from the horrible little people, this way, not that way.' 'Right, let me hit him', 'No'. 'Cos they said something horrible, I went, 'No, they're only small minded people with no brains' [directed at the boys] and they looked at me and went [shocked expression]. I went, 'Anything to say about that mate?' They went, 'No, sorry love' and then walked off and I went 'Bye'. When people wind me up I'm not nice huh.

(Interview One, Hannah, *Embodied Transitions* project)

Hannah's challenge to the boys produced an interaction different from what the laughter should have done. The laughter, like Garland-Thomson's stare (2006), should have made her feel out of place; instead she questioned the boys' right to act as they had. Her challenge refused to accept that her body and its stumble was outside of what should happen in social space. It did not ask for the normate's approval.

The second challenge involves refusing to undertake the work involved in enabling difference to be disguised. Faye, from the *Genetic Journeys* project, was 14 years old and although she did not have a specific diagnosis, had a skin condition of genetic origin that meant she scarred very easily. Her face and other aspects of her body carried numerous scars, which had led to social problems at school. As a result, Faye had been referred to a specialist make-up artist to provide advice on how to disguise her scars. After trying to comply with the complex and very time-consuming labour involved in applying the specialist make-up, Faye decided to reject its use, while still expressing discomfort with the noticeable scarring on her body:

> ...at times I do wish I hadn't fell over and stuff like that 'cos I *hate* my scars so bad. And I can't do anything about them, but really put make-up over them. And I said to a doctor once, and that's all he said. And he referred me to a cosmetologist or something, basically a make-up person. And she spent ages with all like three types of make-up, putting like on each individual scar. And I was like, I'll just use some foundation [laughs] you know, like, it'll save tonnes of time.... So with like actual like, like 'cos you know how that's quite deep like, she was trying to fill them up, there was like one was just a powder, but that was the one you put on after, and the other two were two different colours, but it was so you got your skin tone when you did it.
>
> (One-Off Interview, Faye, *Genetic Journeys* project)

Faye was concerned with the social effects of her scarring, but also ready to find her own way of managing her body in response. Her decision to reject wearing extensive make-up, while still uncomfortable with the visibility of her embodied difference, highlights the space that exists for disabled children and young people to engage with how far they are willing to do the work involved in matching other's ideals of how the body should look.

The third approach to rejecting conformativity moves beyond the choice of passing or accommodation to explore and present embodied difference as something that can be pleasurable. One way this occurs is through the creative ways in which disabled children and young people enact their differences, including through the technologies that at other points are symbols of their bodies as problematic. Frank's mum in the *Enabling Care* project, spoke of how her young son had begun to play with his trachy – a body technology which until then had within his school and his family positioned him as an unwell child who was vulnerable and in need of protection (discussed in more detail in Chapter 3):

> Well, he's started spitting through it which is being discouraged, but that's just the stage, creativity. He was calling it 'super tube' the other day 'cos somebody was saying about, he says, 'I'm sure I could, when we were playing football I could get my tube and I could *blow* that football right in the net!' [laughs].
>
> (Interview Three, Frank's Mum, *Enabling Care* project)

Frank was developing a different relationship to his technology that through his enactment of its connection to him, both blurred the boundary of body and technology, and also produced a different meaning for it. His actions moved it from being a medical technology that kept him alive, to it being a creative and social technology through which he could express himself, show skill and a sense of adventure and fun.

These three brief examples of embodied practice, which did not seek permission or disguise, provide a glimpse of emergent possibilities of non-normative embodiment. What is significant in them is the importance of interaction, of movement, of display, of embodied play in producing such possibilities. In the doing of difference, imaginaries of alternative ways of being and valuing take on a social reality. A disturbance to the usual way of doing things occurs in social space that provides a challenge to normativity, one that refuses to see difference as inherently inferior and other.

Disabled children and young people experience social space as something that questions their belonging. How their bodies fit, or do not fit, the shape of social space; how others make it clear that their way of interacting, their use of technology, is not correct; how they must work (invisibly) towards social norms, leaves their presence contingent on the permission of others. In response, their mode of interacting with people and things is influenced by, at times, attempts to assert belonging through accommodation, and at other times, the right to resist and value their difference. As already indicated, adolescence is a period of hyper vigilance over embodiment that young people generally experience as troubling. The next part focuses on how these balancing acts between disguise, accommodation, and the valuing of difference are influenced by the very particular context of adolescence.

Adolescent embodiment

The disabled young people we worked with in the *Embodied Transitions* project were involved in a series of 'body projects' (Brumberg, 1997) aiming to enact their bodies in ways that were in keeping with markers of appropriate adolescence. At times, such work positioned embodied difference into the background; at other times it was very much brought into the foreground.

Adolescence is a social experience where issues of difference can be particularly marked both in people's interactions with each other and in their body management. Practices associated with 'fitting in' are vital sites of self and other monitoring. Having a body that is different can produce particular challenges; however the nature of those challenges can vary according to other aspects of embodied adolescence. One particular aspect is gender and its association with sexuality, in particular heteronormativity (Gill *et al.*, 2005; Kehily, 2001; Martino, 1999). Various writers in youth studies have emphasised the importance of having the right kind of body in order to display the right kind of masculinity or femininity: 'it is through the acquisition of some bodies or some capacities that certain masculinities become possible' (Hauge and Haavind, 2011: 14). In such accounts, the notion of transition we discussed in Chapter 3 is understood as the 'transformation of subjectivities (i.e. a person's sense of self) from the subject position 'child', which is detached from sexuality, towards constituting themselves as 'adolescent', which means negotiating more explicit intersections of gender and sexuality' (Hauge, 2009: 294). For Hauge, body management in adolescence is closely implicated in the regulatory dynamics involved in young people measuring themselves and others against norms associated with gender and sexuality.

The body is seen as vital in the everyday negotiations young people are involved in, to establish the appropriate femininity or masculinity via the body practices they enact. For example, Swain (2003) discusses how boys become 'some*body*' (original emphasis) through their body practices. Allen (2013: 352) suggests for young men 'the body is a resource' in defining and enacting the masculinities appropriate to the particular spaces they move through and the masculinities that enable privilege and status. Adolescent girls are likewise caught up in such body practices and dynamics of positioning themselves against norms of what is recognised as femininity. For both young men and women, sexuality is important, but remains distinct in the gender norms they are judged against (Hauge, 2009; Richardson, 2010). In keeping with the relational understanding of embodied practice, the role of the body in producing particular gendered and sexualised identities is also one that draws from discourse through the reference point to particular norms (Hauge and Haavind, 2011). So discourses and enacted doings and displays operate together within the identity negotiations young people participate in.

The journals young people produced in the *Embodied Transitions* project display this interaction between embodied and discursive practice. In particular participants were conscious of, and keen to enact, markers of recognisable femininity and masculinity. Kate included several pictures which were of her standing, smiling confidently to the camera. In each image she also was leaning on things around her (e.g. a sink or a door way).

The images made clear reference to norms of adolescent femininity in the care they displayed over appearance (hair swept to one side, nail varnish and make-up, and in Figure 5.1, the pink dress). Femininity was at the foreground of what Kate wanted to present, made possible through the drawing together of what she wore, how she stood and the sink that allowed her to lean in a recognisably 'normal' way. What remains in the background, in order for that discourse to be referenced through her body, is disability. The leaning pose, while necessary for her to stand, could be read as a way of holding the body common to portraiture.

> Well, I mean, obviously I'm leaning on the sink because I can't obviously stand. Well I can now [after surgery] but I don't think, at that point I was just kind of leaning. I don't think that necessarily looks like I'm disabled, because you could just lean against something and that people generally lean against stuff all the time on photos. But not that that would be a problem if it did look like I was disabled, because that's me you know.
>
> (Interview Two, Kate, *Embodied Transitions* project)

Kate was conscious that a possible act of concealment was taking place in the poses she constructed, the enactment of a recognisable version of femininity was

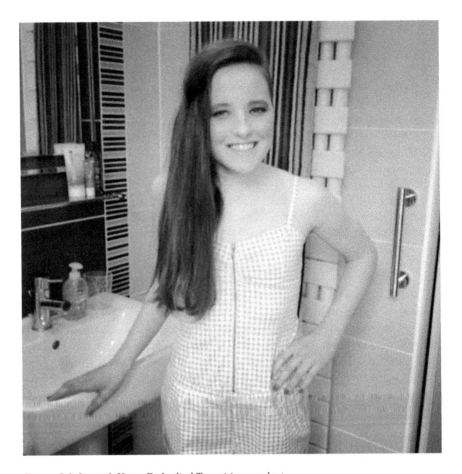

Figure 5.1 Journal, Kate, *Embodied Transitions* project.

deliberate, but she did not want to imply that femininity and disability were intrinsically opposed; however disability's erasure made the visual accomplishment of femininity easier for others to see.

For the young men in the *Embodied Transitions* project, much of their focus was on the link often made between masculinity and strength. For several of the young men sport was the route through which they enacted recognisable forms of young masculinity:

INTERVIEWER: What is it, why do you play rugby?

ANDREW: I've got a good stocky build for it ... And I quite like because I can get all me anger out then just by tackling people.

INTERVIEWER: Yeah?

ANDREW: So people on the pitch that I don't like, I just go straight for them.

INTERVIEWER: Yeah yeah.

ANDREW: With or without the ball.

INTERVIEWER: So you just go for them anyway?

ANDREW: I'm just absolutely psycho when I play rugby.

(One-Off Interview, Andrew, *Embodied Transitions* project)

Here, through a physical and aggressive disability sport, Andrew positioned himself as an assertive young man, able to use sport as a setting where acts of violence could be enacted as acceptable and in keeping with adolescent masculinity. Sport enabled him and others to emphasise the ways in which they were active, in contexts where displays of disability could be barriers to being recognised as masculine:

I think I'm active and sporty, I like doing things, I like doing sports and I like doing activities and that kind of thing.

(One-Off Interview, Daniel, *Embodied Transitions* project)

Like other young men who counterbalance the passivity of office work with time spent in the gym and being involved in body building (Nayak and Kehily, 2008), sport was a way to escape the trap of passivity – particularly important given the presumed passive subject position that comes with disability. Here, disability could be incorporated into a rejection of the passive wheelchair figure, even for those with very limited limb movement, strength and control:

INTERVIEWER: Yeah. And is it important for you, do you think, playing things like that, like Boccia is important?

MATTHEW: [Yeah.]

INTERVIEWER: Yeah? Why?

MATTHEW: Because I want to get better at it.

INTERVIEWER: So you're gonna keep playing then? I mean you said, what did your grandparents say, that you won the championships?

MATTHEW: [Yeah.]

INTERVIEWER: Yeah? Was that at a National level?

MATTHEW: [Yeah.]

INTERVIEWER: Yeah?

MATTHEW: Yes.

INTERVIEWER: That's pretty good. So are you thinking that you'll keep getting better for the future?

MATTHEW: I want to play at the Paralympics.

(One-Off Interview, Matthew, *Embodied Transitions* project)

This produces a strong echo to Hauge and Haavind (2011) and others (Mac an Ghaill, 1994) who argue that the skilful and strong body displayed aesthetically and through enactment is a privileged discursive and embodied site of young heteronormative masculine identity. Masculinity is so tied to the fit, healthy and strong body that the disabled body can appear to be outside of the possibility of it (Gerschick and Miller, 1994; Valentine, 1999). As Valentine discusses, 'a hegemonic masculine style of bodily comportment is about having the freedom to move freely in space and to appropriate it both through physical displays of competence and force, and through having social confidence and a sense of personal security' (Valentine, 1999: 172). Much of the work on the difficulties disability creates for performing masculinity has been undertaken with men with acquired disabilities seeking to rebuild bodies that have fractured the link between their identity and their body practices (Smith and Sparkes, 2005, 2008). While important, such work can be thought of as 'a concern primarily with 'real' men who lost their masculinity, rather than those who were never perceived as masculine in the first place because they had an impairment from an early age' (Shuttleworth *et al.*, 2012: 183).

A prominent narrative, very present in the UK during the 2012 Paralympic Games, is that disability sport symbolises examples of people who overcome their disabilities in order to achieve. This was particularly marked in narratives around young men with acquired disabilities who reclaimed their masculinity through once again becoming strong and powerful in the eyes of 'normal' society (used a great deal amongst athletes who had acquired their impairments through armed conflict). The problem with this narrative is that it supports the notion that body difference itself is outside the realms of masculinity, strength and accomplishment. To be successful despite disability is to say disability and success are essentially in opposition. By looking at the account of one disabled young man in the *Embodied Transitions* project, we want to suggest an alternative to the overcoming story.

Mark, as we know, was an accomplished wheelchair rugby player, recognised at a national level as someone with promise for the future. He had been attracted to the sport due to the very different visual presence it produced around both the disabled body and the wheelchair. This was a body and technology that displayed – for him – strong masculinity and physicality, aggression and significant ability. His disabled body – both what worked and what did not – and the specialist wheelchair he used to participate in the sport – were an intrinsic part of the version of masculinity he created for himself. He rejected wheelchair basketball, like Andrew, in favour of wheelchair rugby because he preferred what he saw as the more aggressive and violent nature of rugby, which turned wheelchairs into assault vehicles:

> For me it would be the big hits, you know it's pretty much illegal anywhere else to bray someone out their wheelchair … I don't really know why I didn't like it [wheelchair basketball], but I just, I really do like rugby, I think it's just, basketball does not hit people and you know I really just do like rugby a lot more better than basketball,… it sounds stupid but you don't really get anywhere else to hit people out of their wheelchair, as well, the team and I think it's the ethic, the team ethic, we all like talk together, which I know that happens in every sport but. I like the big hits and the way team

go on together and just 'cos we're disabled we still have the fire in our bellies to get the big hits in to win.

(Interview Two, Mark, *Embodied Transitions* project)

Mark's participation in sport was the prominent theme in his photographic work; his photographs catalogued his rugby training, team preparations, matches in progress and his life with his team mates (in Chapter 4 we also highlighted the photographs he had taken to show the everyday work involved in building up his body strength). The valued subject Mark displayed was someone who made the disabled body work, there is no distancing from, or disavowal of, disability attempted in his photographs. He was not overcoming the differences in his body, he was using them. The combination of sport with technology and a strong disabled body turned the meanings associated with both the chair and the body from symbols of deficit and inability to something surrounded by a sense of power and accomplishment. The network's meaning was further strengthened through the incorporation of other technologies and scientific practise into it. Due to Mark being identified as someone with a promising future in the sport at a national level, he had been assessed at specialist sport centres seeking to identify how his sporting body could be improved within the arena of disabled sport:

MARK: And you did different tests, that was to see what your body temperature got up to, and this was to see how much oxygen you got into your body. And how much you got out, which is why you needed the mask on.

INTERVIEWER: So why, what kind of results were they looking for?

MARK: To see what the heart rate got up to, as well there's a lot of different disabilities in the sport now, where if there's a spinal injury they can't obviously get the heart rate up to, the injury, they can't get the heart rate up to, I think mine got up to a hundred and twenty. Yeah so that was pretty hard, and this one was your strength, you had to see how long you could hold it for as well.

(Interview Two, Mark, *Embodied Transitions* project)

His photographs included images of the specialist sport medicine monitoring he had had (see Figures 5.2 and 5.3).

At the centre, Mark had been measured for a specialist wheelchair, which, once built, would be fitted to his specific body shape and dimensions and would cost several thousand pounds to make. The technologies associated with sports medicine, the design of a wheelchair just for him, are material artefacts that are far from the sticks or chairs that Mark and others spoke of choosing not to use because they marked them as having bodies that were of less value than other kinds of body. Here the configuration of science, technology and body enables a discourse of value. Mark had a different body worthy of investment in, within a sport which made use of impairment in order to claim recognition in the public sphere as impaired and accomplished. Mark, and the others involved in disability

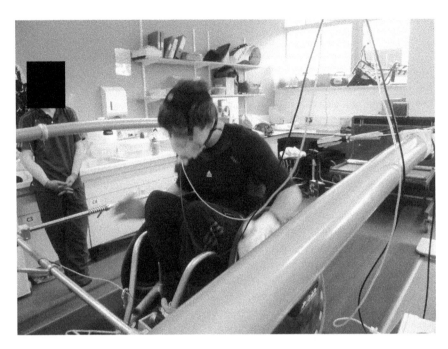

Figure 5.2 Journal, Mark, *Embodied Transitions* project.

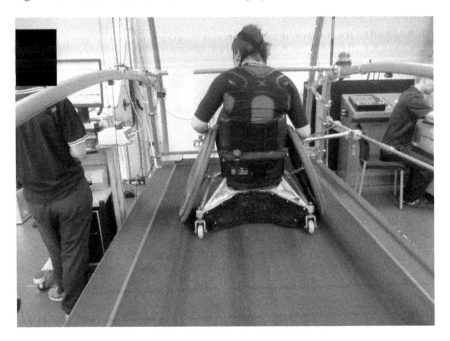

Figure 5.3 Journal, Mark, *Embodied Transitions* project.

sport, created an opportunity to enact a version of masculinity that could be recognised by able-bodied people. It was enabled through their disabled bodies rather than despite of.

There are a couple of caveats to the promise of the relational networks that had developed around and through the body of the disabled sportsman and the associated technologies. These caveats indicate the contingency present in the capacity of this relational configuration of body difference, technological material and scientific measurement to produce the valued disabled masculine body. First, the success of this alternative enactment and narrative requires that others see the figure that is emerging in those relations. Reflecting on why he had prioritised the display of his active, sporting self in his images, Mark acknowledged that he wanted to be recognised as an accomplished disabled sportsman. However, even though to us and him, this self was visible in the images he produced, he acknowledged that people could still look at such images and see the pitiable disabled figure:

> …it depends on who is looking … if you got someone off the street … they'd say 'That's good that they've got into a sport' and 'Bless their cotton socks' rather than 'We beat them, maybe knocked them out the chair, put twenty goals on them and all the play-offs. That's quite strong to do that, how does he continue to do what he does with less functions?' If you're seeing Mo Farah win gold, everybody's 'Yeah get in there', that's represented in the sport. In images [of disabled sport] obviously this is [the same] for me.
>
> (Interview Two, Mark, *Embodied Transitions* project)

Second, the alternative that Mark and others provide, while inclusive of disability within a vision of a valued subject, runs the risk of validating a social norm that a disabled person *should* be busy, active and doing all they can to avoid being the passive victim. This was evident in the embodied figure Mark felt the Paralympics provided a counter to:

> Obviously with the soldiers coming back injured, loads of them seem to play basketball, rugby, volleyball, to make sure they know that there is a sport out there and especially like people see people and think their life is just sitting there, whinging and watching Jeremy Kyle, but you can go and play sport.
>
> (Interview Two, Mark, *Embodied Transitions* project)

To claim public recognition through embodied difference for disabled young people like Mark it appeared to require, particularly as a man, that he be an active disabled young person. While that produces a counterbalance to presumptions of passivity, it appears to run the risk of presenting passivity as the negative trait others have defined it as. In Chapter 3 we highlighted the importance of the trope of self-reliance to the goal of the transition to adulthood. The relational network that emerged in the interface between the disabled sportsman and sports technology made use of embodied difference in its construction; but it also made use of the existing social value placed on being active in order to be recognised.

The body projects associated with the complex world of adolescence were important tasks for young people we have worked with. Through them they sought belonging and identity. At times, disability was incorporated into such tasks, at other times the focus was on making it invisible. Such activity made use of discourse in the articulation of particular claims to gendered normalcy, independence and self-reliance; however without the relational practices that worked on the body to enact and thus shape those discourses, their presence in shaping the boundaries of normalcy would not be possible.

Conclusion

The drawing together of concerns with the social construction of categories of disability with contemporary approaches to understanding how bodies themselves come to matter within a range of social networks is vital to exploring both the limits and potential for situated agency. It captures the prevalence of norms within everyday ways of being and speaking, which curtail opportunities to be different without cost. The significance of everyday rejection to prescribing inequality into the fabric of the everyday comes through in the work required of those who are positioned as different through words and actions to accommodate to others – an accommodation that sets them up to fail through the right retained to judge them as never quite normal enough. That disabled children are already trying to find ways to negotiate their way through to belonging by enacting ordinariness tells us a great deal about the power of the gatekeepers to social recognition. Yet, examining disabled children and young people's embodied practices does also capture ways in which they challenge some of the status quos in front of them. The networks they are active participants in can produce value through, rather than in spite of, difference. They remake themselves, others and technology to open up possibilities for resistant identities that place the emphasis on society to rethink its boundaries and norms.

References

Allen, L. (2013) Boys as sexy bodies: picturing young men's sexual embodiment at school. *Men and Masculinities*, 16(3): 347–365.

Barad, K. (2003) Post-humanist performativity: toward an understanding of how matter comes to matter. *Signs*, 28(3): 801–831.

Barnes, C. (2012) Understanding the social model of disability: past, present and future. In N. Watson, A. Roulstone, and C. Thomas (eds), *Routledge Handbook of Disability Studies*. pp. 12–29. London: Routledge.

Braidotti, R. (1996) Signs of wonder and traces of doubt: on teratology and embodied difference. In N. Lykke and R. Braidotti (eds), *Between Monsters, Goddesses and Cyborgs*. pp. 135–152. London: Zed Books.

Brownlie, J. and Sheach Leith, V.M. (2011) Social bundles: thinking through the infant body. *Childhood*, 18(2): 196–210.

Brumberg, J.J. (1997) *The Body Project: An Intimate History of American Girls*. London: Random House.

Buckingham, D. and Tingstad, V. (eds) (2010) *Childhood and Consumer Culture*. Basingstoke: Palgrave Macmillan.

Butler, J. (1993) *Bodies That Matter: On the Discursive Limits of 'Sex'*. London: Routledge.

Colls, R. (2007) Materialising bodily matter: intra-action and the embodiment of 'fat'. *Geoforum*, 38: 353–365.

Fenton, N.E., Elliott, S.J. and Clarke, A. (2013) Tag, you're different: the interrupted spaces of children at risk of anaphylaxis. *Children's Geographies*, 11(3): 281–297.

Freund, P.E.S. (1988) Bringing society into the body: understanding socialized human nature. *Theory and Society*, 17(6): 839–864.

Freund, P.E.S. (2001) Bodies, disability and spaces: the social model and disabling spatial organisations. *Disability & Society*, 16(5): 689–706.

Garland-Thomson, R. (1997) *Extraordinary Bodies: Figuring Physical Disability in American Culture and Literature*. New York, NY: New York University Press.

Garland-Thomson, R. (2006) Ways of staring. *Journal of Visual Culture*, 5(2): 173–192.

Garland-Thomson, R. (2007) Shape structures story: fresh and feisty stories about disability. *Narrative*, 15(1): 113–123.

Gerschick, T. and Miller, A. (1994) Gender identities at the crossroads of masculinity and physical disability. *Masculinities*, 2: 34–55.

Gill, R., Henwood, K. and McLean, C. (2005) Body projects and the regulation of normative masculinity. *Body & Society*, 11: 37–62.

Goodley, D. and Runswick-Cole, K. (2011) The violence of disablism. *Sociology of Health and Illness*, 33(4): 602–617.

Goodley, D. and Runswick-Cole, K. (2013) The body as disability and possibility: theorizing the 'leaking, lacking and excessive' bodies of disabled children. *Scandinavian Journal of Disability Research*, 15(1): 1–19.

Gottlieb, A. (2004) *The Afterlife Is Where We Come From: The Culture of Infancy in West Africa*. London and Chicago, IL: The University of Chicago Press.

Guntram, L. (2013) 'Differently normal' and 'normally different': negotiations of female embodiment in women's accounts of 'atypical' sex development. *Social Science & Medicine*, 98: 232–238.

Hammer, G. (2012) Blind women's appearance management: negotiating normalcy between discipline and pleasure. *Gender & Society*, 26(3): 406–432.

Hauge, M.I. (2009) Bodily practices and discourses of hetero-femininity: girls' constitution of subjectivities in their social transition between childhood and adolescence. *Gender and Education*, 21(3): 293–307.

Hauge, M.I. and Haavind, H. (2011) Boys' bodies and the constitution of adolescent masculinities. *Sport Education and Society*, 16(1): 1–16.

Hennessy, R. (1993) *Materialist Feminism and the Politics of Discourse*. New York, NY: Routledge.

Hoffman, M. (2013) Bodies completed: on the physical rehabilitation of lower limb amputees. *Health*, 17(3): 229–245.

Hughes, B. (2009) Wounded/monstrous/abject: a critique of the disabled body in the sociological imaginary. *Disability & Society*, 24(4): 399–410.

Imrie, R. (2001) Barriered and bounded places and the spatialities of disability. *Urban Studies*, 38(2): 231–237.

Imrie, R. (2013) Shared space and the post-politics of environmental change. *Urban Studies*, 50(16): 3446–3462.

Kehily, M.J. (2001) Bodies in school: young men, embodiment, and heterosexual masculinities. *Men and Masculinities*, 4: 173–185.

Kirk, S. (2010) How children and young people construct and negotiate living with medical technology. *Social Science & Medicine*, 71(10): 1796–1803.

Kitchin, R. (1998) 'Out of place', 'knowing one's place': space, power and the exclusion of disabled people. *Disability & Society*, 13(3): 343–356.

Lee, N. and Motzkau, J.F. (2011) Navigating the bio-politics of childhood. *Childhood*, 18(1): 7–19.

Mac an Ghaill, M. (1994) *The Making of Men. Masculinities, Sexualities and Schooling*. Buckingham: Open University Press.

Marks, D. (1999) Dimensions of oppression: theorising the embodied subject. *Disability & Society*, 14(5): 611–626.

Martino, W. (1999) 'Cool boys', 'party animals', 'squids' and 'poofters': interrogating the dynamics and politics of adolescent masculinities in schools. *British Journal of Sociology of Education*, 20(2): 239–263.

Mayall, B. (1996) *Children, Health and the Social Order*. Buckingham: Open University Press.

Mol, A. (2002) *The Body Multiple: Ontology in Medical Practice*. Durham, NC: Duke University Press.

Mor, S. (2006) Between charity, welfare, and warfare: a disability legal studies analysis of privilege and neglect in Israeli disability policy. *Yale Journal of Law and the Humanities*, 18: 63–136.

Nayak, A. and Kehily, M.J. (2008) *Gender, Youth and Culture*. Basingstoke: Palgrave Macmillan.

Parens, F. (ed.) (2006) *Surgically Shaping Children: Technology, Ethics and the Pursuit of Normality*. Baltimore, MD: The Johns Hopkins University Press.

Paterson, K. and Hughes, B. (1999) Disability studies and phenomenology: the carnal politics of everyday life. *Disability & Society*, 14(5): 597–610.

Richardson, D. (2010) Youth masculinities: compelling male heterosexuality. *The British Journal of Sociology*, 61(4): 737–756.

Shildrick, M. (1999) The body which is not one: dealing with differences. *Body & Society*, 5(2–3): 77–92.

Shildrick, M. (2005) The disabled body, genealogy and undecidability. *Cultural Studies*, 19(6): 755–770.

Shildrick, M. (2012) Critical disability studies: rethinking the conventions for the age of postmodernity. In N. Watson, A. Roulstone and C. Thomas (eds), *Routledge Handbook of Disability Studies*. pp. 30–41. London: Routledge.

Shuttleworth, R., Wedgwood, N. and Wilson, N.J. (2012) The dilemma of disabled masculinity. *Men and Masculinities*, 15(2): 174–194.

Smith, B. and Sparkes, A.C. (2005) Men, sport, spinal cord injury, and narratives of hope. *Social Science & Medicine*, 61(5): 1095–1105.

Smith, B. and Sparkes, A.C. (2008) Changing bodies, changing narratives and the consequences of tellability: a case study of becoming disabled through sport. *Sociology of Health & Illness*, 30(2): 217–236.

Snyder, S.L. and Mitchell, D.T. (2001) Re-engaging the body: disability studies and the resistance to embodiment. *Public Culture*, 13(3): 367–389.

Söderström, S. (2009) The significance of ICT in disabled youth's identity negotiations. *Scandinavian Journal of Disability Research*, 11(2): 131–144.

Staples, J. (2011) At the intersection of disability and masculinity: exploring gender and bodily difference in India. *Journal of the Royal Anthropological Institute (N.S.)*, 17: 545–562.

Swain, J. (2003) How young boys become somebody: the role of the body in the construction of masculinity. *British Journal of Sociology of Education*, 24: 299–314.

Thomas, C. (2002) The 'disabled' body. In M. Evans and E. Lee (eds), *Real Bodies*. pp. 64–78. Basingstoke: Palgrave.

Thomas, C. (2004) Disability and impairment. In J. Swain, C. Barnes, S. French and C. Thomas (eds), *Disabling Barriers – Enabling Environments*. pp. 21–27. London: Sage.

Thomas, C. (2007) *Sociologies of Disability and Illness. Contested Ideas in Disability Studies and Medical Sociology*. Basingstoke: Palgrave.

Valentine, G. (1999) What it means to be a man: the body, masculinities, disability. In R. Butler and H. Parr (eds), *Mind and Body Spaces: Geographies of Illness, Impairment and Disability*. pp. 167–180. London: Routledge.

Wendell, S. (1996) *The Rejected Body: Feminist Philosophical Reflections on Disability*. New York, NY: Routledge.

Williams, S., J. (1999) Is anybody there? Critical realism, chronic illness and the disability debate. *Sociology of Health & Illness*, 21(6): 797–819.

Zitzelsberger, H. (2005) (In)visibility: accounts of embodiment of women with physical disabilities and differences. *Disability & Society*, 20(4): 389–403.

6 Making family

Introduction

We have explored how social interactions and social space are important to the production of social monitoring and othering of disabled children and young people. When children are in social space they are often in the company of family. Within the relationships that shape disabled children and young people's lives and identities, family is of key importance. An important theme of disability studies work on family has been to challenge the dominance of accounts in health and social policy that speak of the burden of having a disabled child that families have to manage (McLaughlin, 2012). This work has been rejected for the medicalised approach it takes to understanding disability (as a personal and familial tragedy) and identifying the problems and solutions (aiding families to cope better with the burden of that tragedy). Disabled children are part of their families, not just something for their families to manage. A wealth of research within disability studies has captured the varied experiences of families with disabled children. Key findings include that much of the 'burden' that families discuss they connect to the battles they fight with social and health care services to receive adequate and appropriate care and support (Heaton *et al.*, 2005; McLaughlin, 2006; Preston, 2006; Read, 2000). They also see another source of 'burden' in their lives being the social observation they must manage. The staring that Garland-Thomson (2005) identified as an important mechanism in situating the disabled person as other is a stare that is also directed at their families as complicit in the emergence of their disturbing presence in social space. Across both disability studies and medical sociology, the interest in how the staring dynamic draws in family has led to the concept of stigma being used to explore the difference disability in childhood makes to family life.

As indicated in Chapter 1, stigma is a concept we find valuable because it provides an interactionist way of understanding how normal ways of doing things enable others to be set apart because of their lack of fit with those standard practices. It also enables us to consider how that setting apart does not just happen to the person, but also to those associated with them. Given our focus on relational practice and networks an approach that draws in the importance of both everyday interaction and relationality is clearly something we would find helpful. However, in looking at the concept, we also think it is important to do so critically, acknowledging some of the problems others have found in the ways in which it has been adopted in research examining disability and family life. Therefore, while making use of the concept in this chapter, we also highlight some problems with it and draw in three other approaches that help to examine disability and family more broadly. First is sociological work examining how families are involved in societal dynamics of othering that are associated with the value placed on different class positions. This work aids us by highlighting social categories other than disability which can place a family and its members under social scrutiny. Second is social anthropological and sociological work on family which considers how family relationships are socially and culturally formed. This work helps explain how the making and doing of familial relationships inform how people respond to disability, particularly its categorisation by medicine. Finally, we make use of feminist work that connects the practices of care found in families to the production of recognisable family forms. This work enables us to explore how one aspect of care practices associated with disability is the opportunity they provide to refute the lack of value a family with a disabled child is assumed to have.

By bringing these approaches together we are able to do several things. First, we indicate how disabled children and young people are participants in their families; part of the relational network that shapes the boundary of what a family is and who its members are. Second, we relate the importance of the broader social location of a family to how disability comes to matter and the availability of resources available to them to care for their child and raise them as they would wish. Finally, we can consider how families are located within the dynamics of monitoring we are interested in across the book.

Stigma

Social stigma, from an interactionist perspective, is a form of social monitoring that influences the social position, in particular patterns of marginalisation, that disabled children and those associated with them experience. Goffman's ([1963] 1990) work is where most accounts of stigma and disability, particularly in the context of family, begin. As a symbolic interactionist, Goffman recognised the importance of embodiment to the categorisation of types of being and interacting as deviant and stigmatising. Norms of how the body should look and act police acknowledgement in social interactions. In his account, embodied difference is not inherently stigmatising but becomes so in interactions whereby the meanings generated between people get attributed to differences that break with perceived bodily norms. As Smith (2000: 85) states, Goffman was not concerned with the fact of stigma per se, but how different contexts construct different things as stigmas. A difference becomes a stigma when it is deemed by others to be discrediting, and as it creates a discrepancy between a person's assumed 'virtual' social identity and their 'actual' social identity (Goffman, [1963] 1990: 12).

Writers seeking to explore the social experiences of families with disabled children use the notion of stigma to consider the 'costs' of being associated with someone who differs from expectations of how a child should behave and look – what Goffman referred to as 'courtesy stigma' (Ryan, 2005; Ryan and Runswick-Cole, 2008). Jones (2013: 30), drawing from her own experiences of growing up alongside a brother diagnosed with learning disabilities in the US in the 1960s and 1970s notes: 'Families that include someone with a disability are often re-situated in the margins of society, set slightly askew from other families due to the unfamiliar and the unknown'. Kwang Hwang and Charnley's (2010) research with siblings of disabled children in Korea shows how their experiences of marginalisation through association were influenced by cultural understandings of disability as something that shames a family. This is because it is a punishment placed on the family for previous sins. Francis, in a useful discussion of stigma research in different socio-cultural locations, produces a helpful summary:

> caring for a child with disabilities alters one's place in the prevailing social order, undermines claims to normalcy, and disrupts valued relationships and identities. The stigma can be felt or enacted – parents sometimes experience isolation and shame because they anticipate negative labelling, while, in other cases, rejection and discrimination are directly manifest in interaction.
>
> (Francis, 2012: 928)

In our research, family members have recounted multiple examples of social interactions that place them and their child/ren into the category of 'other' (McLaughlin et al., 2008). Those with children with visible physical impairments experience the pity and charity response that both infantilises the child (for example by not speaking directly to them) and presents the parents or siblings as heroic sacrificial carers (Landsman, 1999). Families with children whose embodied difference is not immediately recognisable to others as a socially or medically validated disability can find themselves questioned for their use of support such as car parking reserved for disabled people, or why their child looks funny or wears those fancy glasses. Finally, children whose behaviour, whether recognised within disability categories or not, falls outside of social norms can lead to questions about the appropriateness and response of parents (particularly mothers) and whether it is fair on others to bring such children into public space (Blum, 2007). A key reason parents seek medical answers to why their children are different is to manage this range of social interactions (Gray, 1993, 2002). It also links to the parental quest we highlighted in Chapter 4 to normalise their children's bodies and behaviours to be more in keeping with their social worlds now and into the future (Kittay, 2006; Leiter, 2004).

The question in responding to and understanding why families with disabled children face such social monitoring is whether an account that relates it to stigma, particularly stigma produced by embodied difference, is sufficient. It is clearly a component influencing why people display and enact such discomfort and awkwardness, but there are some problems in relying on it solely. The various problems researchers have raised each relate to the need to question whether it is disability that is always the troubling factor generating the 'stickiness' in the social interaction (Davis, 1961).

First, we need to question whether it is the child or the parent who is the subject of social scrutiny. Francis (2012) argues that it is important to distinguish more clearly the difference between courtesy stigma – the problems of being associated with a disabled child – and parental blame – the problems associated with being seen as the cause of a child's problems. In scenarios where the disability is not socially recognised or medically defined, the focus of the social judgement can revolve around the parents, particularly the mother, as being inadequate in managing their child (Green, 2003, 2004). In this circumstance the stigma dynamic is different: in one case the judgement is targeting the child, and the parents experience the problems of being associated with that child. In the latter scenario the judgement is shared between child and parent and is less about association and more about targeting blame towards parents. In Francis's research (2012) she found dynamics of parental blame were less likely (but not removed entirely) when children had been diagnosed with biomedical classifications of disability, which worked to remove blame from the parents and onto other factors such as genetics. Normalising the child then is a strategy for managing courtesy stigma, while medical diagnosis is a strategy for managing parental blame. Both problems come from social monitoring, but the subject, and therefore the solution, is different.

Dynamics of parental blame are more likely to play out when other social factors outside of disability appear within the social interaction, in particular other sources of discredit such as class, age, and marital status. In stigma accounts of how families with a disabled child become 'disabled families' via their association with that child, there is a risk that disability is seen in isolation to other ongoing dynamics of judgement and monitoring that families may already experience. Courtesy stigma implies a tranquil, happy family of social acceptance and integration, unsettled by the presence of disability within its life. Instead a disabled child is as likely to enter a family where dynamics of judgement are already in play and which will influence how that family and that child is read. To enable us to consider the intersection of social categories of discredit we turn to contemporary sociological work on class and valuing.

Regimes of value

A useful way to think about the significance of multiple social categories to social monitoring and policing is to draw from the sociologist Bev Skeggs's concept of 'regimes of value' (2011). Skeggs uses this concept, developed from years of ethnographic research in working class communities in the UK, to make visible the power that accepted norms in a society have and their location in material and cultural inequalities between classes. Such regimes of value inform who is recognised as appropriate subjects through the judgements made about how people live and what they articulate as their moral outlook. Skeggs, whose approach is closely influenced by Bourdieu (1989), prioritises class but also incorporates embedded inequalities around gender, race and ethnicity, and sexuality into her analysis (unfortunately she has not incorporated an interest in disability into her work). For her, it is the middle class subject who is recognised as valuable through their acquisition of capital, their focus on individual success and their (apparent) lack of need for support from others, in particular the state. In contrast, working class subjects and their families are assumed to be lacking; in the UK an influential political narrative around such families is to position them as 'troubled families' (Levitas, 2012), marked by multi-generational patterns of unemployment, criminality, and uncontrolled reproduction. In response, Skeggs (2001) suggests that those tarred by such narratives produce their own counter narratives – often by valuing the very relationships said to define their lack of respectability.

From this perspective, attempts to acquire a medical diagnosis for a child or any other family member is an attempt to acquire credibility from a socially valued source of knowledge and status; one given more value in society than other ways of defining the sources of the child's problems. Callard *et al.* (2012: 281) have explored such attempts to look to medicine to absolve social blame within the field of genetics, in particular genetic diagnoses of schizophrenia. Genetic diagnosis 'has the capacity to reorganise a family's telling of its own history to itself and to others – through genealogies that are produced through scientific knowledge as well as (re)imagined kin relations'. In the context of existing explanations of schizophrenia (themselves a product of psychiatric medicine) most notably the trope of the bad mother, genetics can be used to suggest no person is to blame. However, Callard *et al.* also caution that such talk does not necessarily silence such existing explanations; the power of the figure of the bad mother is hard even for genetics to dispel.

We have witnessed similar attempts to escape the category of the bad mother in the *Genetic Journeys* project; it was notable that mothers who seemed most focused on finding an explanation that took the blame away from them shared vulnerable social locations that placed them under social scrutiny. Such mothers were 'lone mothers', or 'mother with children from multiple partners' – forms of family relationship rarely given value and respect in UK society, particularly if also associated with a class position thought of as working or lower class (Lawler, 2002). When asked to describe her class position, one lone mother noted: 'I'm classed as a single parent, benefit scrounger with two disabled children' (Interview One, Lucy's mum, *Genetic Journeys* project). Lucy's mother found that she had to challenge various assumptions about her mothering skills in order to have the possibility that there was something medically wrong with her children acknowledged:

I had a three year battle, going through Learning Disabilities Team saying I was molly coddling them, there was nothing wrong with them.... 'Cos at first they said, 'oh you just want her to be disabled.'... All sorts of accusations come out, you know, 'you're just making it up.' Or you get people in the street saying, 'you're doing it for the DLA [Disability Living Allowance] benefit'.

(Interview One, Lucy's Mum, *Genetic Journeys* project)

Connor's mother, another lone parent, found herself under considerable scrutiny by medical professionals when her baby did not gain weight:

I kept on saying he's not growing, he's not putting on any weight. This was probably at about a year old, about eleven months, and they just kept on saying, 'ah, just give him more calories.'... They weren't doing anything to start with, and then it was, when he was like really, really, *really* tiny, they were like, 'we'd better have another look.' When he was about *three* that was. Yeah, great that!

(Interview One, Connor's Mum, *Genetic Journeys* project)

For these two mothers, genetic explanations offered an opportunity to redefine their child's problems as medical and in so-doing produce a counter-balance to the argument that the source lay in their irresponsibility. Therefore, disability was not the stigma being managed or escaped. Instead they sought a medical category of disability, in order to escape another form of stigma they experienced, one captured by Skeggs and Loveday's (2012) notion of 'regimes of value'. Their family setting was already, through social monitoring, defined as lacking value. Their aim was that a medical, in this case genetic, validation that their child was disabled, rather than a product of their imagination or poor parenting, would produce a better narrative to situate the family as a whole. Accounts of courtesy stigma do support the notion that parents seek medical validation to redefine the child as having a condition, but the focus remains on understanding this process as an attempt to solve the problem of being associated with a problematic child (read as unruly, naughty), rather than the problems the child has in being associated with the family and the broader regimes of value being in that family places the child within.

Making family

Stigma accounts focus on how the world around the family shape it. In the process another weakness is the lesser attention given to how the family world provides its own response to disability, which may escape notions of stigma and othering. Going back to Kwang Hwang and Charnley's (2010) research with siblings of children with diagnoses of autism in Korea, they found even in contexts where the stigma of such a label was particularly high, the siblings carved out a life for themselves that included their disabled sibling and which expressed 'ordinariness' as much as it managed 'difference'. Taylor (2000), drawing on long term ethnographic research with an extended family in the US whose members had been diagnosed with a range of different learning disability and physical disability categories, explores how the family had developed shared meanings of who they were that were distinct to the categories others had placed them within. There was recognition of difference, of a need for support; however, the categories used by institutional and societal others did not produce senses of shame or othering, which they felt they must manage. Their differences had become incorporated into their cultural world and to some degree sanitised from the attributions others might give them. Based on what he had learnt from his time with the family, Taylor (2000: 89) concludes: 'Theories of disability seem to take stigma for granted and proceed to examine how people manage it, whether through passing, denial or resistance ... they do not necessarily account for the experiences of people embedded in different family worlds'. Making a similar observation, Gray (2002: 737) suggests some of the problems with the use of the concept of courtesy stigma, lies in the narrowing of the dynamic to the particular interactions occurring between families and others, in the process excluding the 'broader biographical nature of their [the family's] relationship with their child'. For Gray (2002: 737) the broader 'biography' remains the 'identity as the parent of a child with a disability'. In contrast, we would argue there is a need to expand our understanding of the social dynamics around othering and stigma to include the broader biography of the family and the social, cultural and economic contexts that inform that biography (Davis and Salkin, 2005). Extending how we understand the relationship between family life and the narratives of disability that emerge for and from a child or young person can be supported by drawing from contemporary work on family and kinship from across sociology and anthropology.

There is now a substantial body of work examining the social production of family ties and understandings of kinship (Franklin and McKinnon, 2001; Jamieson, 1998; Smart and Neal, 1998). As with our own work, this research brings together an interest in narrative and practice into how it explains how family formations emerge, are maintained and recognised/mis-recognised. In terms of narrative, it examines how people come to define certain relationships as familial; the influence of broader socio-cultural values attached to family in the formation of those ties – in particular narratives of naturalness, biology and reproduction – and the ways in which family ties can be retold within new imaginaries, counterpoints to existing framings (Edwards, 2000, 2005). As touched upon in Chapter 4, we may (sometimes but not always) be born into relationships already defined as familial, but those relationships require framing and placement, particularly if anything in those relationships begins to deviate from social expectations of what a family is and looks like. Haimes (2003) speaks of the narrative work families do to integrate a child into a family network when their route into that set of relationships has been different, for example through adoption or via the use of reproductive technologies such as IVF. Carsten (2004) makes an important distinction between family as something 'given' to us, and also something that is 'made'.

Practice comes in through examination of the importance of people 'doing' family in cementing norms via rituals such as christenings, marriage, parents' evenings at school, or the family meal (Morgan, 1996). The specifics of those rituals will vary across time and place, but what appears common is the need to participate in them in order to show oneself as within appropriate ways of being a family. Finch (2007: 67) extends this idea by suggesting it is the display of, as well as the participation in, the practice that enables 'individuals, and groups of individuals, [to] convey to each other and to relevant audiences that certain of their actions do constitute 'doing family things' and thereby confirm that these relationships are 'family' relationships'. In an argument similar to Haimes (2003), Finch proposes that the more one's family relationships appear to deviate from certain norms, the more important it is to participate in such recognised displays of family life. For example, Taylor (2009), in research with lesbian and gay households with a child in the UK, argues that the participants appeared to approach everyday rituals such as the 'family meal' and participating in their child's schooling as important ways they could validate that they were families 'just like anyone else'.

One form of display is via artefacts that symbolise those experiences, connections and people of value within a kinship network. Such artefacts are made meaningful through their connection to the person associated with them: the clothing kept of a child when they were a baby; the lock of hair kept of someone who has died; or formal material such as the display of a family tree (Finch and Mason, 2000; Williams, 2004). Paramount within such artefacts are images of family, whether displayed in photo albums, or on the walls of the 'family home', or in more contemporary possibilities, such as digital photo albums either shared within the family or with others online. These images become meaningful through the narratives people tell of them; narratives that are both particular in their reference to specific people and events that have occurred within that family, but also more broadly social in their references to the wider narratives that are available within particular socio-cultural locations to signify family (Gilmore, 2001). The stories told of the loving grandmother, or the hardworking father, or the brave disabled child, draw from existing scripts of what families look like, pointing also to the possible boundaries to kinship-making that people develop their sense of family within (Kellas, 2005; Mason, 2004; Misztal, 2003; Smart, 2007). Finch (2007: 78) defines family narratives as 'stories which people tell to themselves and to others about their own family relationships, which enable them to be understood and situated as part of an accepted repertoire of what 'family' means'. This has strong echoes with historian Gillis's (1996) influential distinction between the families we 'live with' and those we 'live by'; that is the myths and stories that act as windows into what is socially valued as family. The narratives that indicate the families we live by reflect 'a family's values, culture, and its collective meanings' (Kellas, 2005: 367). Therefore, storytelling provides versions of what family is, and who does and does not belong, interpreted by those within the family and outside of it. Children can be active in such storytelling and displays of family; in our research when children were given journals, pictures and stories of family were (perhaps unsurprisingly) dominant and vivid (see later in this chapter).

Work is now emerging that takes these approaches to kinship-making to explore how family ties are made and remade in the context of disability, providing at times new ways to both do family and have that recognised by others as still valued ways of both being different and a family. For example, Rattray (2013), in ethnographic work he undertook with a wheelchair rugby team in Ecuador, highlights how narratives of family – spoken of as '*segunda familias*' or 'second family' – emerged within the team in their respect and care for each other, in contexts where few others were offering such recognition. There may be struggles over ensuring that such alternative family formations built around disability are recognised by others as valuable, but in their practices and displays, possibilities of different ways in which people can do family that challenge societal norms are seen. This includes new ways to frame and practice care that provide a counterbalance to privatised and sacrificial narratives. Such narratives also provide ways to enable and acknowledge how a disabled child can, through their presence, play a role in remaking family ties.

Part of the presence a child has is embodied, something the anthropologist Kelly has explored through her US ethnographic research examining the production of meanings from and about disabled childhoods, within contexts of family life. Her key claim is that meanings of impairment and parenting inform each other:

> Impairment is experienced and made meaningful through particular systems of meaning and parent identities, demonstrating the interplay between personal engagement with notions of materiality and embodiment and the ongoing social and cultural contexts in which parents, as agents of impaired children, act and interact.
>
> (Kelly, 2005: 187)

Practices of care that emerge around impairment alter how people think of themselves as parents and what parenting constitutes. It also leads them to think differently about impairment as they work towards the social inclusion of their children as part of their newly-defined role. In part, this can be framed as a response to the stigma they identify in such social spaces; however, it also emerges out of the re-imagining of family they are participating in, and which their child is also a participant in. Definitions of impairment, practices of care and formations of parenting identity come together through narrative and enactment, produced across a range of 'private' and 'public' spaces to produce ongoing sets of meanings and values around disability and the recognition of the child as a social subject.

Across our projects we have seen multiple ways in which existing family biographies and practices influenced how a child's embodied differences were both understood by others and enacted by them. We have already touched on genetics as a form of medical knowledge and categorisation, which may be turned to in attempts to absolve family members of blame for the problems their child has. However, such attempts are tricky to pursue, because they also can become the source of an equally troubling story about a family's value (as noted in Chapter 4): in particular that they are the source of bad blood. Genetics could then be used as further proof that a family, their kin, including their children, are without value, right through to their genetic make-up (Carsten, 2007; Sachs, 2004). Understanding how genetics can inform whether a family is recognised as valued is dependent on how it becomes incorporated into existing family narratives, in particular stories around inheritance (Edwards, 2005; Rapp and Ginsburg, 2001).

The interplay of kinship stories with genetics was often articulated in the *Genetic Journeys* project (McLaughlin and Clavering, 2011). Families brought existing narratives around family history, particularly of ill-health and disability, into their exchanges with geneticists and then their incorporation of genetic narratives into this ongoing familial history (Latimer, 2013). For example, genetics and kinship narratives and symbolic artefacts were brought together in the attempts Kyle's parents made to claim a social space for their version of family, in particular a space for children that could enable them to be seen as valued social actors. While both parents had difficult histories, it was the maternal side that was under the most scrutiny. The mother described her history as one marked by periods of being in care, of her siblings being in care, of absent and changing parental figures, of unstable familial structures and roles (in the past, siblings had referred to her as mum) and significant material insecurity and deprivation. She also spoke of a wish to remove herself and her immediate family from her biological relatives; however, she was unsure she could. Almost as proof that her background is problematic, the genetic service had told her that the genetic variation they had identified in their son had come from her:

MUM: So I don't know if, back in my past, or my family's past, that we had a member of the family like the way my son [the child referred to the genetic service] is. [Sighs] But having found out that we might have to have the blood test to figure out how far back it does go. It has thrown up quite a few questions for me … with me being put in Child Services, and having so many different schools, I've had a poor education that's why I am re-doing my Maths and English. So maybe that's part of it as well. [Pause] With my learning difficulties, and *my* behaviour has rubbed off, passed onto them. Because they can get rather aggressive can't they? Especially Kyle, 'cos he gets frustrated, quite a lot, when he doesn't get his way, or when he feels like he's not understood.

(One-Off Interview, Kyle's Mum and Dad, *Genetic Journeys* project)

Her past is now present – genetically – in her son, emphasising for her the permanence of her connection to her biological family. This relational connection, by being emphasised by genetics, risks concretising an association that stigmatises via the lack of social value and material and cultural capital associated with those ties – more so than does the son's disability. The narratives available to her about her background offer little to protect her or her 'immediate family' from social judgement as being one of those problem multi-generation families with problem children they cannot take care of. Due to the problematic connection being kinship rather than, or more than, disability, it is within kinship that any challenge to that way of the family being read and positioned must occur.

This occurred through a couple of narrative associations of value being made, one which made use of non-biological ties, another via biological ties; both of which were evidenced through visual artefacts. The first association was to a friend of Kyle's mother (who had been a friend of the now-deceased maternal grandmother). The friend was described as the mother's adopted mother and as being, along with her husband and children, her core family. The family's home, in an economically deprived area, was full of photos, both on the wall and in albums. Much of their interview was spent going through them. The mother's wish to escape her 'real' family was marked by their complete absence within these visual artefacts of family, which they valued as being the most important possession they had. Instead, the displays of family included the adopted mother as central to the family she was making with her husband and children:

MUM: But to me, family is important and if I didn't have these two [pointing to photograph of her 'adopted mum' and her adopted mum's husband], I would rather not have my biological family, I would rather have these two and the family that I've got now. And that would be my life.

(One-Off Interview, Kyle's Mum and Dad, *Genetic Journeys* project)

The second association was to emphasise how much the children took after their father and his side, rather than her and her side. The photographs were used to display the visual similarity between the children, their father and their dead paternal grandmother (Hirsch, 2002; McLaughlin and Clavering, 2012):

MUM: Yeah, so dad's eyes ... they used to think that was our daughter when she was little, it wasn't, it's her dad

...

and there [points to photograph of daughter] ... Looks like her grandmother ... When she was younger, [points to photograph of the paternal grandmother as a young girl] that's his mam

...

See, they don't look anything like me, the only thing they've got off me is my hair.

(One-Off Interview, Kyle's Mum and Dad, *Genetic Journeys* project)

The mother here draws from a recognised narrative of family – visual resemblance – displayed in photographic artefacts to counter other narratives of problematic kin, which trouble her children's social position. Disability is part of the dynamic here, but the broader social location and tales of her extended family are more significant in the children's marginality. Her response indicates the power of existing narratives of family to be a factor in social marginalisation, but also the spaces that exist to offer alternative narratives in response.

Our projects have also provided testimony of ways in which practices of doing/making family can be vehicles through which embodied difference is incorporated into what and who a family is; consciously doing so in a way that makes use of embodied difference as a source of both family practice and evidence of value. One way fathers and sons enact their bonds is in shared interests in sport (Fitzgerald and Kirk, 2009). This can either be through participation in sport, or it can be through shared support of a particular team or type of sporting activity. The birth of a disabled son can disrupt that recognised gendered family practice, one response we have seen is for disabled boys and young men to retain an interest in sport as evidence of their belonging to a family. In our *Embodied Transitions* project, male (and a few female) participants spoke often of their strong interest in both watching and participating in sport (usually rugby or football); this was often narrated as something they did with dads and brothers. They also spoke of times they felt excluded from the family routines, which occurred around the consumption of sport, or participation in it. The prominence of sport in the accounts is influenced by the significance of team sports in the North of England, particularly to the display and enactment of masculinities.

Paul, first in his SPARCLE interview as a young child, and in both interviews with us, spoke of the importance of football to him, his non-disabled twin brother and his family. The one picture of himself he put in his journal was him wearing an England football strip. As a child he went along to the same football club his brother was a member of. While he was allowed to train with the other boys and play in friendly games, when it was league matches he was not allowed to play. In his first interview with us he noted his continued interest in football, but that unlike his brother he was unable to play in a 'normal' team:

PAUL: like me brother, he plays for a football team. And sometimes I think 'Ah, I wish I could have done that', but I can't, like just a normal one.
INTERVIEWER: What do you mean normal football team?
PAUL: Why just like a football team, just people without problems and that.
(Interview One, Paul, *Embodied Transitions* project)

By the time of his second interview with us, Paul had started to play in a disability football team. However, it was evident that one aspect of what made football meaningful to him was that it was an interest and embodied practice he shared with his brother. Pointing to a picture of his brother in his journal, Paul commented:

And this is me twin brother. When we were younger we used to play, play football and that, but now we we're like season ticket holders, to get see [favourite team] home matches which is, which is good to go to.
(Interview Two, Paul, *Embodied Transitions* project)

The segregation of sport into 'normal' and 'disabled' sport created problems for Paul to enact his connection to others in his family; highlighting to him the way he differed from his brother, emphasising a theme across his interviews that his brother was normal and he was not. While watching football with his brother and dad was an activity they could share and enact their shared familial interest, the problems he found when trying to participate in sport meant an opportunity to enact that shared activity was lost.

However, we also saw instances where disability, rather than being a threat to the carrying out of such displays of family connection, could become incorporated into it. Such incorporation leaves the gendered consumption and participation of sporting activity untouched as a symbol of appropriate family connection and enacted masculinity. However, by disability being drawn into its enactment, the boundaries of what makes the activity an expression of family connection and masculinity can be expanded. This was seen at its most expressive in the family life of Mark in the *Embodied Transitions* project. Mark, as we have already discussed, was a wheelchair rugby enthusiast. Much of his young masculine identity was embedded in his participation in the sport, and his father was his close ally in this. His father took him to all matches, and was heavily involved in the team. Mark chose to focus on his participation in wheelchair rugby in his photo journal, and his father took all the photographs for him. The photos, the father's involvement in taking them, and his participation in the team point to this activity being a vital symbolic display of Mark's identity both as a young man, and a young man within a family which saw sport as an important shared interest (what little spare time Mark and his father had away from wheelchair rugby, they spent watching their local professional football team play). The pride his family took in Mark's success was a display both of their recognition of his achievements and of disability being a part of who he was and who they were as a family.

Family relations are made and remade in the stories people tell of them and the practices they enact to display to others that they are not only family, but family of worth and value. Disabled children can trouble some of that family labour, but families are likely to be involved already in ongoing processes to maintain their social position and validity. Drawing the child into their accounts and practices of family incorporates them into ongoing approaches to enacting value. One such practice that is central in identifying and validating family is care.

Care practices

That families provide care is a family narrative and practice that is readily recognised. Feminist sociologists in the Global North have examined both the narratives and practices of care to highlight the ways in which care is not something that should be understood as a self-evident property of families (Barrett and McIntosh, 1991; Campbell and Carroll, 2007; Donzelot, 1997). Instead it is a product of historical, political and economic structures that have solidified boundaries between the private and the public, alongside everyday local negotiations within families of who does what, informed by those structures (Finch,

1989; Finch and Mason, 1993). Practices of who cares and who should care are culturally informed norms and values, framed within specific cultural locations and made meaningful through how they are enacted within families (Rapp and Ginsburg, 2001). The cultural specificity of family care practice is visible through the differences in how care is framed and done in different cultural locations. For example, research in Asian countries (and migrants from those countries living in the Global North) emphasise the significance of concepts of filial piety and obligation within the degrees to which different people within families express and then practice caring roles. Filial piety implies that children owe life-long obligations to their parents (rather than asserting their independence from them). Daughters (and daughters-in-law) should enact that care through the provision of it (including having older parents within their households when they are adults raising their own children), while sons' enactment is focused on the provision of financial support (Funk, 2012; Won, 2012).

We can think of care as an important regime of value that families, particularly those without material sources of value, practice and display in order to acquire or retain acceptability (Skeggs, 1997). If one role of care is to enable the enactment of valued practices and identity, then it is likely to influence the form of care that is produced and the way in which it is narrated. Looking at work on care and disability, various writers have highlighted how valued care norms influence the ways in which narratives of sacrifice are formed around caring for a disabled child as both a valued practice for families, and for women in particular (Garro and Yarris, 2009; Landsman, 1999; Larson, 1998; Traustadóttir, 1995). Prussing *et al.* (2005: 588), in a narrative analysis of the accounts of US mothers' approaches to caring for their disabled children, suggest that tales of motherly sacrifice are a way to contest 'prevalent cultural explanations that frame a child's disability as a mother's personal failure ... or a divine punishment'. Garro and Yarris (2009) argue, in a visual ethnography of parental care of disabled children also in the US, that parents prioritise displaying both practices of self-sacrifice (particularly mothers), but also practices geared towards still seeking to prepare that child for a successful independent and individual adulthood, as a way of positioning both them and their child as acceptable within societal narratives of successful parenting and childhood.

Family and the care it provides was a theme that understandably came up often in both the childhood interviews and the variety of work the disabled young people did with us in the *Embodied Transitions* project. A common theme was to recognise the importance of the care their families, in particular their mothers, provided for them as something they really appreciated and valued (see Figure 6.1).

Sean was a participant who had taken a great deal of care over the production of his journal, bringing together photographs of himself and family, images downloaded from the web, clip art and typed text which explained his views on different things. An important theme in the journal was how much his family meant to him and how much he appreciated the care they provided. In response

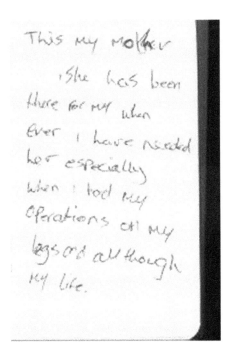

Figure 6.1 Journal, Paul, *Embodied Transitions* project.

Note
The text reads 'This is my mother [alongside was a picture of Paul's mother], she has been there for me whenever I have needed her, especially when I had my operations on my legs, all through my life.

to a photography task that asked him to represent who or what supported him, he produced the image and text shown in Figure 6.2.

In the care and work Sean took over the production of the photography material it appeared to matter to him a great deal that he could display his life and those around him in ways that would be recognised by others as being of value. When discussing the image in his photo elicitation interview, he explained further:

> ...got a brilliant family, absolutely brilliant family, couldn't ask for a better family ... I mean me parents take us to hospital appointments, they take us to physio, they're always there, me mam sat beside me hospital bed when I've needed her...

> (Interview Two, Sean, *Embodied Transitions* project)

The version of family that comes across in the participants' accounts was their absolute dependability, a belief that they would always be there, something they felt particularly important to them given the challenges their disability produced

- If it wasn't for the love, support,
  understanding and acceptance of my parents
  that I have received/ receive now and in the
  past I would not be the person I am and I
  wouldn't lead such a great life. My parents
  take me to physio and hospital appointments
  etc.

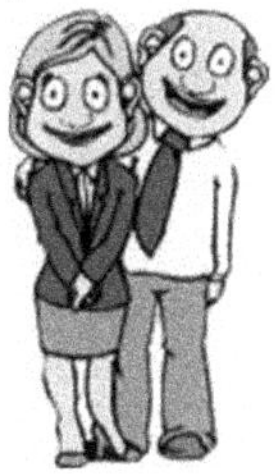

Figure 6.2 Journal, Sean, *Embodied Transitions* project.

(or more correctly the challenges created by the medical treatment of their embodied differences and the problems created by an unwelcoming social world):

SARA: They [family] give you support don't they.
INTERVIEWER: Support, in what ways do they give you support?
SARA: Like say if I'm going for operations they'll be there. Obviously if you go for an operation you're in pain, so they'll be there to give you moral support and hugs and everything really, they'll be there for you. Or if you're having a bad time then they'll just sort of be there…. It's just a family thing really.
(Interview One, Sara, *Embodied Transitions* project)

Friends, as well as family, were incorporated into such representations of the value and importance of care. Kate, in response to the task about who or what supported her, shared a picture of herself with her best friend (produced as a Selfie via the built-in camera of her laptop). In her journal, alongside the image, she gave an explanation as to why (see Figure 6.3).

While the narrative of the importance of her friend to Kate broadens the family narrative to include friends, it is still a recognisable and familiar narrative, which links female friendship to a language of care and support. Her account shares the same gendered account found in many of the accounts of family care participants produced; it is mothers, and here a female friend, who are singled out as the people who will always be there for you. By drawing from gendered recognisable narratives, the choice of text and image link the personal expression to the public values of family care practice: that which displays what a proper family is (regardless of blood ties) against norms of value which enables us to read such relationships as family or akin to family (such as a close friend).

Task 8 – Someone or Something that supports me:

This is me and my best friend ▓▓▓▓. I have chosen her for this task because she really is everything you could wish for in a best friend. I know it's a cliche but she truly is always there for me whenever I need her to be, and always says the right thing to cheer me up or make me feel better. Whether i've got a cold, or get stressed with exams or whatever, I can always rely on her for a hug, with out fail. She makes me laugh, and brightens up dull times, and when it is dull, we can cry together, and feel better straight afterwards. We've had our "ups and downs" but, only very occasionally, and in the past couple of years, not at all. We really do never fallout, we just seem to know each other so well, and any ups and downs we had when we first met five years ago, after starting secondary, have allowed us to understand each other more and more, and now, she provides unfailing support for me, just when I need it.

Figure 6.3 Journal, Kate, *Embodied Transitions* project.

These images and text speak to a Global North ideal of family that is easily recognisable. In these extracts, family is recognisable both through the standard ties of kinship – biological mother and father and other siblings, alongside extended family – and through the gendered practices and displays of care they enact. Such gendered framings tell us a number of things about how caring narratives and practices are informed by the broader social world (Prussing et al., 2005). It is understandable that their accounts draw from recognised repertoires of what a family is, whose responsibility it is do what, and that they discuss such practices in ways that naturalise and privatise them. This is the dominant narrative they see around them in the social world: care is the province of those close to you, family and, to some degree, friends. It is also possible to suggest that they are participants, like parents, in a narrative enterprise seeking both value for themselves as worthy of care, and their families, particularly mothers, as worthy of respect through their commitment and care towards their child.

However, while the participants were proud of what their families did for them, they were also conscious that the labour involved in that care came at a cost to their families and to them. For their families, their worry was the toll the physical nature of that care meant:

INTERVIEWER: And what kind of things make you feel sad?
CRAIG: Well my mam hurts herself sometimes and that makes us sad, 'cos like, she's got a little bit of a hernia there, I hope she doesn't hear that, she's got a little bit of a hernia and when she has to lift us sometimes it hurts her, so that makes me sad.

(SPARCLE Childhood Interview, Craig, *Embodied Transitions* project)

Their concern with the impact of their care on their mothers was an important driver to the embodied practices they undertook in order to be able to do things by themselves and have less reliance on family. The cost to themselves was as they moved into adolescence; the visibility of this care was understood as a visible barrier to them articulating and enacting the adult independence we have discussed in Chapter 3 as a key aspiration for them. The visibility of the care they received from family, beyond that expected as people move into adolescence, they perceived as a social marker of their difference from other young people. There are two implications for them and for how we think about how the care needs of disabled young people are socially and politically positioned, which are important to recognise. First, there was little remark from participants of the role of the welfare state in providing the care they had received from family when young, or would have to manage without as adults. There was little sense of an entitlement narrative, which produces an expectation and request that social welfare should be a provider of care and enabler of independent living in the context of disability (Morris, 1993). The loss of this entitlement narrative narrows the possible alternatives to family care and generates greater emphasis on the individual to care for themselves and produce a body that can be cared for by the individual. Second, visibly receiving care from family that others apparently did not need once an adolescent is not judged as normal. However, if we think of the material and cultural capital which adolescents in particular class positions receive as a form of care, and which is vital to their apparent 'independence', then it is clear that it is only certain types of care that are judged as problematic. The ability some have to provide material and cultural capital for their children, combined with narratives of self-sufficiency that disguise the importance of that form of care, creates inequality. It is this inequality that fuels the efforts young people put into body projects that seek to make them respected independent adults.

Conclusion

The language of burden and sacrifice that is found in some research on disabled children and young people and family risks constructing the child or young person as something 'the family' have to manage. Such a narrative recreates the sense that the child is an external force and threat rather than a part of that family life. An important counterbalance to the burden account is instead to see the child as a participant in reimagining the family's identity, future and aspiration. Stigma has captured the work families do to respond to the social interactions and scrutiny they experience that define them, including their disabled members, as out of place in the public sphere. However, stigma has limits in capturing how family life comes to inform the lives and identities of disabled children and young people, including their role in shaping how family influences their life and how they influence the lives of the families they live in.

The link between broader existing narratives of what family is and the narratives families then tell, clearly has a political dimension. The approved scripts that indicate what families should be and how others seek to prove themselves against them via display of the appropriate practices, indicate the making of family ties and sense of belonging is not simply an issue of choice and preference. Indeed, it is important to think of the inequalities that can exist around which families are seen more easily as acceptable and what patterns of marginalisation may be found in such processes. The enactment of care, both in private and in public, and the incorporation of disability into family practices, are important re-imaginaries that push for more expansive recognition of different forms of family identity and formation. The work that families do to be recognised as valuable highlights the blurred nature of the private and public boundary. It also takes us into questions of citizenship, which we would now like to explore as a way to draw the themes of the book together. We do so by working through the relationship between monitoring and regulation and difference and identity for the opportunities disabled children and young people have to be citizens.

References

Barrett, M. and McIntosh, M. (1991) *The Anti-Social Family*. London: Verso.

Blum, L.M. (2007) Mother-blame in the Prozac nation – raising kids with invisible disabilities. *Gender & Society*, 21(2): 202–226.

Bourdieu, P. (1989) *Distinction: A Social Critique of the Judgement of Taste*. London: Routledge.

Callard, F., Rose, D., Hanif, E.-L., Quigley, J., Greenwood, K. and Wykes, T. (2012) Holding blame at bay? 'Gene talk' in family members' accounts of schizophrenia aetiology. *Biosocieties*, 7(3): 273–293.

Campbell, L.D. and Carroll, M.P. (2007) The incomplete revolution – theorizing gender when studying men who provide care to aging parents. *Men and Masculinities*, 9(4): 491–508.

Carsten, J. (2004) *After Kinship*. Cambridge: Cambridge University Press.

Carsten, J. (2007) Constitutive knowledge: tracing trajectories of information in new contexts of relatedness. *Anthropological Quarterly*, 80(2): 403–426.

Davis, C.S. and Salkin, K.A. (2005) Sisters and friends – dialogue and multivocality in a relational model of sibling disability. *Journal of Contemporary Ethnography*, 34(2): 206–234.

Davis, F. (1961) Deviance disavowal: the management of strained interaction by the visually handicapped. *Social Problems*, 9: 120–132.

Donzelot, J. (1997) *The Policing of Families*. Baltimore, MD: Johns Hopkins University Press.

Edwards, J. (2000) *Born and Bred: Idioms of Kinship and New Reproductive Technologies in England*. Oxford: Oxford University Press.

Edwards, J. (2005) 'Make-up': personhood through the lens of biotechnology. *Ethnos*, 70(3): 413–431.

Finch, J. (1989) *Family Obligations and Social Change*. Cambridge: Polity Press.

Finch, J. (2007) Displaying families. *Sociology*, 41(1): 65–81.

Finch, J. and Mason, J. (1993) *Negotiating Family Responsibilities*. London: Routledge.

Finch, J. and Mason, J. (2000) *Passing On: Kinship and Inheritance in England*. London: Routledge.

Fitzgerald, H. and Kirk, D. (2009) Identity work: young disabled people, family and sport. *Leisure Studies*, 28(4): 469–488.

Francis, A. (2012) Stigma in an era of medicalisation and anxious parenting: how proximity and culpability shape middle-class parents' experiences of disgrace. *Sociology of Health & Illness*, 34(6): 927–942.

Franklin, S. and McKinnon, S. (eds) (2001) *Relative Values: Reconfiguring Kinship Studies*. Durham, NC: Duke University Press.

Funk, L.M. (2012) 'Returning the love', not 'balancing the books': talk about delayed reciprocity in supporting ageing parents. *Ageing & Society*, 32: 634–654.

Garland-Thomson, R. (2005) Staring at the other. *Disability Studies Quarterly*, 25(4): http://dsq-sds.org/article/view/610/787

Garro, L.C. and Yarris, K.E. (2009) 'A massive long way': interconnecting histories, a 'special child', ADHD and everyday family life. *Culture, Medicine and Psychiatry*, 33: 559–607.

Gillis, J.R. (1996) *A World of Their Own Making*. Boston, MA: Harvard University Press.

Gilmore, L. (2001) Family frames: photography, narrative, and post-memory. *Signs*, 27(1): 283–286.

Goffman, E. ([1963] 1990) *Stigma: Notes on the Management of a Spoiled Identity*. London: Penguin Books.

Gray, D.E. (1993) Perceptions of stigma: the parents of autistic children. *Sociology of Health & Illness*, 15(1): 102–120.

Gray, D.E. (2002) 'Everybody just freezes. everybody is just embarrassed': felt and enacted stigma among parents of children with high functioning autism. *Sociology of Health & Illness*, 24(6): 734–749.

Green, S.E. (2003) 'What do you mean "what's wrong with her?"': stigma and the lives of families of children with disabilities. *Social Science & Medicine*, 57: 1361–1374.

Green, S.E. (2004) The impact of stigma on maternal attitudes toward placement of children with disabilities in residential care facilities. *Social Science & Medicine*, 59(4): 799–812.

Haimes, E. (2003) Embodied spaces, social places and Bourdieu: locating and dislocating the child in family relationships. *Body and Society*, 9(1): 11–33.

Heaton, J., Noyes, J. and Sloper, P. (2005) Families' experiences of caring for technology-dependent children – a temporal perspective. *Health and Social Care in the Community*, 13(5): 441–450.

Hirsch, M. (2002) *Family Frames: Photography, Narrative and Post-memory*. Cambridge, MA: Harvard University Press.

Jamieson, L. (1998) *Intimacy: Personal Relationships in Modern Societies*. Cambridge: Polity Press.

Jones, M.M. (2013) The 'othered' sister: family secrets, relationships, and society. *Review of Disability Studies*, X(2&3): 30–40.

Kellas, J.K. (2005) Family ties: communicating identity through jointly told family stories. *Communication Monographs*, 72(4): 365–389.

Kelly, S.E. (2005) 'A different light' – examining, impairment through parent narratives of childhood disability. *Journal of Contemporary Ethnography*, 34(2): 180–205.

Kittay, E.F. (2006) Thoughts on the desire for normality. In E. Parens (ed.), *Surgically Shaping Children: Technology, Ethics and the Pursuit of Normality*. pp. 90–110. Baltimore, MD: The Johns Hopkins University Press.

Kwang Hwang, S. and Charnley, H. (2010) Making the familiar strange and making the strange familiar: understanding Korean children's experiences of living with an autistic sibling. *Disability & Society*, 25(5): 579–592.

Landsman, G. (1999) Does God give special kids to special parents? Personhood and the child with disabilities as gift and as giver. In L.L. Layne (ed.), *Transformative Motherhood: On Giving and Getting in a Consumer Culture*. pp. 133–164. New York, NY: New York University Press.

Larson, E. (1998) Reframing the meaning of disability to families: the embrace of paradox. *Social Science & Medicine*, 47(7): 865–875.

Latimer, J. (2013) *The Gene, the Clinic and the Family*. London: Routledge.

Lawler, S. (2002) Mobs and monsters: independent man meets Paulsgrove woman. *Feminist Theory*, 3(1): 103–113.

Leiter, V. (2004) Dilemmas in sharing care: maternal provision of professionally driven therapy for children with disabilities. *Social Science & Medicine*, 58: 837–849.

Levitas, R. (2012) There may be trouble ahead: what we know about those 120,000 'troubled' families. *Poverty and Social Exclusion in the UK*, Policy Response No. 3: www.poverty.ac.uk/system/files/WP%20Policy%20Response%20No.3-%20%20'Trouble'%20ahead%20(Levitas%20Final%2021April2012).pdf

Mason, J. (2004) Personal narratives, relational selves: residential histories in the living and telling. *Sociological Review*, 52(2): 162–179.

McLaughlin, J. (2006) Conceptualising intensive caring activities: the changing lives of families with young disabled children. *Sociological Research Online*, 11(1): www.socresonline.org.uk/11/1/mclaughlin.html

McLaughlin, J. (2012) Understanding disabled families: replacing tales of burden with ties of interdependency. In N. Watson, C. Thomas and A. Roulstone (eds), *Routledge Companion to Disability Studies*. pp. 402–413. London: Routledge.

McLaughlin, J. and Clavering, E.K. (2011) Questions of kinship and inheritance in pediatric genetics: substance and responsibility. *New Genetics and Society*, 30(4): 399–413.

McLaughlin, J. and Clavering, E.K. (2012) Visualising difference, similarity and belonging in paediatric genetics. *Sociology of Health and Illness*, 34(3): 459–474.

McLaughlin, J., Goodley, D., Clavering, E.K. and Fisher, P. (2008) *Families Raising Disabled Children: Enabling Care and Social Justice*. Basingstoke: Palgrave Macmillan.

Misztal, B. (2003) *Theories of Social Remembering*. Milton Keynes: Open University Press.

Morgan, D.H.J. (1996) *Family Connections*. Cambridge: Polity Press.

Morris, J. (1993) *Independent Lives*. Basingstoke: Macmillan.

Preston, G. (2006) Families with disabled children, benefits and poverty. *Benefits: Journal of Poverty and Social Justice*, 14(1): 39–43.

Prussing, E., Sobo, E.J., Walker, E. and Kurtin, P. S. (2005) Between 'desperation' and disability rights: a narrative analysis of complementary/alternative medicine use by parents for children with Down's syndrome. *Social Science & Medicine*, 60(3): 587–598.

Rapp, R. and Ginsburg, F. (2001) Enabling disability: rewriting kinship, reimagining citizenship. *Public Culture*, 13(3): 533–556.

Rattray, N. (2013) Wheelchair basketball teams as 'second families' in Highland Ecuador. *Review of Disability Studies*, IX(2&3): 92–103.

Read, J. (2000) *Disability, the Family and Society: Listening to Mothers*. Buckingham: Open University Press.

Ryan, S. (2005) 'People don't do odd, do they?' Mothers making sense of the reactions of others to their learning disabled children in public places. *Children's Geographies*, 3(3): 291–305.

Ryan, S. and Runswick-Cole, K. (2008) Repositioning mothers: mothers, disabled children and disability studies. *Disability & Society*, 23(3): 199–210.

Sachs, L. (2004) The new age of the molecular family – an anthropological view on the medicalisation of kinship. *Scandinavian Journal of Public Health*, 32(1): 24–29.

Skeggs, B. (1997) *Formations of Class and Gender*. London: Sage.

Skeggs, B. (2001) The toilet paper: femininity, class and mis-recognition. *Women's Studies International Forum*, 24(3/4): 295–307.

Skeggs, B. (2011) Imagining personhood differently: person value and autonomist working-class value practices. *Sociological Review*, 59(3): 496–513.

Skeggs, B. and Loveday, V. (2012) Struggles for value: value practices, injustice, judgment, affect and the idea of class. *British Journal of Sociology*, 63(3): 472–490.

Smart, C. (2007) *Personal Life*. Cambridge: Polity Press.

Smart, C. and Neal, B. (1998) *Family Fragments*. Cambridge: Polity Press.

Smith, G. (2000) *Erving Goffman*. Abingdon: Routledge.

Taylor, S.J. (2000) 'You're not a retard, you're just wise': disability, social identity, and family networks. *Journal of Contemporary Ethnography*, 29(1): 58–92.

Taylor, Y. (2009) *Lesbian and Gay Parenting: Securing Social and Educational Capital*. Basingstoke: Palgrave Macmillan.

Traustadóttir, R. (ed.) (1995) *A Mother's Work Is Never Done: Constructing a 'Normal' Family Life*. Baltimore, MD: Paul H. Brookes Publishing Co.

Williams, F. (2004) *Rethinking Families*. London: Calouste Gulbenkin Foundation.

Won, S.-Y. (2012) Gendered working-time arrangements and their policy implications: Korean experiences. *Time & Society*, 21(3): 285–307.

Part IV

Implications

7 Embodied and relational citizenship

We draw the book to a close by exploring what the varied forms of monitoring and surveillance we have detailed mean for disabled children and young people's citizenship – now and into their adult futures. Before we do so we will first summarise how sociological understandings of citizenship have opened up due to long term shifts in political context and changes in theoretical conception (Turner, 2000a; van Steenbergen, 1994). These changes in understandings and context are helpful for thinking about both the limits and possibilities for disabled children and young people as citizens.

Under the significant influence of Marshall's (1950) account of what he saw as the evolution of different components of citizenship, citizenship is now widely explored as something more than formal rights provided for the recognised citizen of the state. He proposed that through history you can see the emergence of broadening rights of citizenship. First came civil rights that guaranteed individuals protection in law over things such as property. Then came political rights via the right to vote and to participate in the electoral system. Finally, in the twentieth century, came social rights that gave people entitlements to certain things from the state, in particular the protection of the welfare system, which enabled them to participate in society. Marshall is now challenged for the aspects of history he excluded in order to tell a linear account, and for his unacknowledged basis in a particular Western history (Fraser and Gordon, 1994; Turner, 2000b). It is not surprising that various writers have highlighted that this expansion of rights has been less linear and inclusive than his narrative provides for. Feminists (Dietz, 1987; Kofman, 1995; Yuval-Davis, 1991) have highlighted that all these rights have been something women have had to fight for long after their establishment for (some) men. When we think of disability and the still recent history of institutionalisation beyond the time he argued that the trinity of civil, political and social rights had been established in law, politics and welfare, it is clear that this expansion did not include disabled people and continues to be fought for.

During the decades immediately after Marshall's text, in the shifting political culture of the 1960s and 1970s, as social groups marginalised from those apparent entitlements challenged their exclusion, the components of citizenship broadened out again to include questions of cultural identity and recognition

(McLaughlin *et al.*, 2011). Alongside asking for formal rights, groups called for greater recognition of different ways of living and being. Within the politics of race, women's rights and sexuality rights, there was an exploration of who the imagined holder of rights was (Yuval-Davis, 2011). Groups asked not just to be included, but to challenge the particular version of citizenship available. As a consequence of the emergence of identity politics, work on the regulatory dynamics of citizenship now includes asking what people are required to enact as particular templates of personhood in order to be recognised as legitimate. Garland-Thomson's (2011) misfits are those who are judged by others as incapable of matching normative citizenship ideals. These ideals are encapsulated in representations and narratives that shape our understandings of citizenship; but they are also embedded in a range of institutionalised and embodied practices. As Turner (2000b: 2) argues 'Citizenship may be defined as that set of practices (juridical, political, economic and cultural) that define a person as a competent member of society, and which as a consequence shape the flow of resources to persons and social groups'. Although the identity politics of the 1960s and 1970s is associated, to a degree, with an expansion in who and what could be included in citizenship and its practices (for example in relation to sexual liberation), in the era of neo-liberalism, economic austerity, welfare reduction and global capitalism some speak of a shrinking back in normative possibilities within citizenship. A return to that mythical figure of the independent, self-reliant worker (Hindess, 2002).

To draw this back into our concern with disabled childhoods, in this chapter we will examine two different aspects of the citizenship possibilities for disabled children and young people. First is the influence of prevalent notions of who is the good adult citizen. In the book we have documented the considerable efforts made by disabled children and young people to get ready to become a particular kind of adult. In doing so, they are working towards the recognised template about what citizenship entails and requires. We will propose that this implies that one condition on being recognised as an adult citizen is conforming to a particular way of being one, which is exclusionary towards embodied difference. This generates regulatory dynamics that are productive of particular embodied practices. Second is the question over whether alternative ways of thinking about citizenship could be used to advocate for disabled children and young people being thought of as citizens now, rather than just in the future. We will explore whether opening up citizenship to the everyday practices of participation and belonging in society can – when present – provide opportunities for disabled children and young people to have a say in their lives, and to have those lives valued. Within this we again make use of relationality as a way to think differently about who has the capacity to be citizens.

Conditions on citizenship

Disability studies, at its inception, drew the clear parallel between the focus in European countries in the nineteenth century and the first half of the twentieth century on the industrial worker and the absolute forms of social control that occurred for disabled people (Oliver, 1996). Other disability scholars have argued that modernity's celebration of the rationality of 'man' produced an ideal type of citizen recognised for 'his' intellect, cognitive powers and moral maturity, which in turn justified the exclusion of disabled people (and women and others) from rights and citizenship (Silvers and Francis, 2005). However, we now live in a different era – Global North societies are less reliant on the physical strength and stamina of the factory worker as modes of working have changed and become increasingly technologically-mediated. We have also seen the emergence of disability politics and disability rights legislation, in the UK, but also in other countries across both the Global North and South. These legal and political challenges have led to de-institutionalisation, increasing the presence of disabled people in various societal spaces, including mainstream education. Together, these changes imply less total social marginalisation of disabled people, as the shift away from institutionalisation has generated greater space for wider social participation. There is much to recognise and celebrate in such changes. However, drawing from the different experiences and dynamics discussed in the book, we would like to argue that access to citizenship rights for disabled children and young people remains conditional and that such dynamics of conditionality are targeted towards the mind-body and the individual. Therefore, dynamics of marginalisation may have changed and to some degree lessened, but nevertheless it is important to question the types of regulatory dynamics that now target the disabled young mind-body and to posit alternatives to these modes of governmentality.

Embodied conditionality

Conditionality is a term that is used to highlight the ways in which access to welfare rights has become increasingly conditional on proving one's eligibility. (Dwyer, 2004a, 2004b). It signifies the increased significance of means testing and limitations, such as time restrictions within social security provision, and the increasing requirements on those receiving benefits to prove they continue to qualify. However, here we would like to take the question of conditionality into the domain of thinking about disabled children and young people and their families. In particular, to think about the conditionality that appears evident in the way in which they are thought of as present or future citizens, concentrating on embodied aspects and the influence notions of normality have on prescribing what kind of citizens disabled young people should be trying to become. This focus is influenced by work within embodiment studies that highlights the governmentality of bodies through social policy (Bacchi and Beasley, 2002; Enright, 2011). The dynamics of regulation – both by the self and by institutions – are important aspects of how we can connect embodiment to the conditionality of citizenship in the contemporary era.

Conditionality can be broadened out to also refer to the institutional, social and cultural dynamics that use notions of being normal as vital to being recognised as a valued subject. Again medicine (and other institutions, as we shall see) plays a role in constructing the boundaries of normality and the access to recognition it provides. Various disability writers have questioned medicine's focus, as discussed in Chapter 4, on intervention and therapy in order to enable a child to appear and function more normally. From everyday practices such as trying to keep a child walking, to more invasive and 'cosmetic' surgeries to make a child's face appear more normal, such actions imply a condition is being placed on social acceptance. One of the troubling features of such interventions, from a disability studies perspective, is the involvement of parents in approving and at times advocating them. Some have argued that parents' participation in such actions on their child's body suggests that not only is there conditionality embedded in a child's social acceptance, but that the conditionality of public recognition finds its way into the intimate familial sphere as relationships there are informed by those same values and judgements (Ouellette, 2010).

Medicine is not the only institution seeking to mould the child's body closer to normality. As we highlighted in Chapter 3, education is a key sphere where children are judged against norms of normality and where acceptance into the spaces of education can be conditional on their closeness to such measures. Education seeks to contain (sometimes via medicine's help through the provision of pharmaceuticals to dampen down a child's 'excessive' behaviour) and exclude embodied practices read as disruptive to the social order of that space. Such controlling practices draw both the present and the future together in ways that require us to consider their significance for the possible imaginaries of citizenship for disabled children and young people. The desire to contain bodies in educational spaces is tied to key objectives of education: creating the suitable citizens of the future able to enact the correct social behaviours and responses expected of them once they move into the adult world. Cohen and Morley (2009: 164) see the 'action of the examination, surveillance, and normalising gaze focused and acting upon the body' in education as explicitly linked to its goal of 'making, creating and enforcing assumptions about the citizenship potential of the child'. On the one hand, it could be argued that if disciplinary techniques enable a child to participate in education and gain the skills that will enable them to be social participants as adults, then this is a good thing. On the other hand, however, if such techniques instead focus on creating docile and conforming minds-bodies then they reinforce a disciplinary conditionality placed on being included in society. Understanding the significance of the work done to shape children into particular kinds of social participants and future citizens requires situating such everyday practices into a wider state logic of making the right kinds of people.

As highlighted in Chapter 1, scrutiny of children is a long-established state practice of the Global North, with the key aim of producing future productive adult citizens. From the historical emergence of limits to children and young people being present in the workplace, through to the provision of access to education, a guiding influence has been embedding in children the right kinds of values and approaches to responsibility that will see them make the appropriate contribution to society as adults (Cockburn, 2013). It is far from new that families have been incorporated into the making of good citizens through the responsibility 'encouraged' on them, differentially focused at mothers, to produce and appropriately raise the right kinds of children (Williams, 2008). Such children are also expected to be healthy; in the nineteenth century era this meant healthy enough to work and to fight in order to protect the nation (Lewis, 1980). In the contemporary era it means they must match the requirements of the independent, autonomous neo-liberal citizen. This then clearly generates issues for children and young people whose minds-bodies differ from that healthy norm. It is the gap between what is understood as the good citizen, and living in a mind-body that apparently makes it difficult to become that person, which influences the institutional and, at times, parental focus on intervening, monitoring and surveying a child's development. This is done in the hope that the gap can narrow between who a child is supposed to be becoming and the child themselves.

In Chapters 4 and 5 it was clear it was not just medical actors or parents who sought such modifications, it was also children and young people themselves. Those chapters drew out the intensive and constant work disabled young people themselves do to try to ensure their bodies can be thought of as entitled. We have shown how the young people in the *Embodied Transitions* project placed great significance on working their bodies towards ideals of normality. It is clear from Chapters 3 and 5 that it is normality rather than some imaginary heroic that frames these young people as deficient and which they seek to acquire. The additional work this gives them, and others' whose bodies differ from such ideals, creates distance between them and citizenship. Their bodies become entitled through the display of accomplishment and normality, through not displaying the work that lies behind it and through minimising/hiding those elements of bodily difference that continue to exist (Charmaz, 1995, 2002; Scully, 2010). Others have found connections between attempts to gain or regain valued citizenship status and the body work of disabled people. For example, Galvin (2003) argues that adults who become disabled seek to get back into work, not just to have an income, but to ensure they still have a publicly-valued identity as a contributing member of society. In contemporary narratives that emphasise opportunity, resilience and the valuing of self-accomplishment, competing moves from being an option to being a requirement. This move hides the social reality that the rules of the game benefit some more than others, and rejects the need for a safety net for those who fail against those expectations and measures of success.

The important successes of the disability movement, given new visibility and critical voice by the impact of austerity economic conditions and welfare minimisation, alongside agendas of inclusion in areas such as education, imply a greater space for disabled young people to be participants in society. However, Chapter 3 highlighted the micro dynamics of exclusion still at play, which should lead us to caution against assuming we now exist in an expansive space of belonging and recognition. What may have changed is a move from the secrecy and silence of confinement in institutions, to individualised micro-practices of self-monitoring and self-disciplining, which require significant labour by those now 'allowed' to belong, producing contingency to that inclusion and inequality between those who must work to be good enough to be included and those who remain within the privilege of normality. This has echoes with Fitzpatrick's (2001) argument that the eugenics of the new genetics is not equivalent to the state eugenics of the Nazi period (and other state practices of eugenics in the US, UK and Scandinavia). Instead, he argues, we are in an era where eugenics operates through neo-liberal discourses and practices of choice – placing individuals at the heart of the process, but also requiring them to do the work involved in judging who should be present. Likewise the 'micro exclusions' Holt *et al.* (2012) identified in contemporary education spaces said to be 'inclusive' highlight the complexity of contemporary disputes and boundaries of what kinds of bodies get to belong in varied spaces. The maintenance of social order and the prioritisation of certain values and ways of being that fit with state interests are still shaping the lives of disabled young people; it is how this occurs that has changed. As Shildrick (2005: 33) argues 'Faced with the profound unintelligibility of anomalous embodiment, what has changed is not the problematic, but the way in which it is managed'. The advocacy of children and young people themselves striving to become normal speaks to the governmentality present in contemporary society and biomedical possibilities. This brings to the fore the link between body modification and questions of citizenship as it symbolises the conditions placed on recognition and participation in society: doing all you can to be as normal as possible. What this means is that disabled people have been released from institutions, but offered instead a 'normal life' they must work towards. Making recognition conditional on normality leaves unacknowledged the possibility that the differences said not to fit could instead be thought of as valued diversities, which expand, rather than restrict, human and social possibilities. What this means for Shildrick is that society offers a minimalist version of hospitality through which disabled people are granted certain things and are expected in return to be grateful.

As highlighted earlier, one way to capture the ways in which embodiment, materiality and discursive framings produce conditionality within citizenship opportunities for disabled young people is Garland-Thomson's (2011) notion of the 'misfit'. It is a concept that 'lodges injustice and discrimination in the materiality of the world more than in social attitudes or representational practices, even while it recognises their mutually constituting entanglement' (Garland-Thomson, 2011: 593). This concept echoes much of what we have sought to do in the book, challenging the over-emphasis on discourse in accounts of both the social production of disability and the importance of notions of normality in setting the boundaries of who is allowed to be present in social space. Garland-Thomson (2011: 594) explores the 'co-constituting relationship between flesh and environment' in order to capture the 'encounter between bodies with particular shapes and capabilities and the particular shape and structure of the world'. This both acknowledges the ways in which the built environment produces many barriers that are disabling, but also the interplay of that environment with dynamics of recognition and mis-recognition that also generate disability. What disabled people lack in social space is the 'material anonymity' of ordinariness. Within attempts to fit in she sees both a cost and a benefit we have witnessed in our work with young people: 'the benefit of fitting is material and visual anonymity, the cost of fitting is perhaps complacency about social justice and desensitising to material experience' (Garland-Thomson, 2011: 597).

Of course, disabled young people are not the only young people under such scrutiny and required to prove their worth in order that they can be present in different public spaces and locations. Instead, what we have discussed here in relation to embodied differences framed as disability is part of wider policing dynamics of difference that target young people from a variety of social backgrounds not valued in the contemporary neo-liberal state (MacDonald, 1997). Such policing is embodied, in both the segregation enacted on those young people – the way in which young people gathering in public space is seen in itself as a threat – and in the way in which young people can be targeted because of the way in which their bodies are viewed as different – due to skin colour or body size or dress. An important theme in youth studies is how various aspects of social policy are undermining the citizenship possibilities for young people, for example, increasingly criminalising young people, particularly those from ethnic minority backgrounds and working class locations (Garland, 2001; Jamieson, 2012; Muncie, 2006). Youth governance has a wide net, antagonistic towards a growing range of youth embodiment and identity.

What we have highlighted so far are a number of ways in which there are significant material, cultural and institutional barriers to disabled young people being citizens now or in the future. The way welfare, medical and educational structures respond to different embodiment requires an emphasis on deficiency and lack to obtain support, which brings with it a projection of the child or young person as problematic due to their inability to be normal – according to norms others have set. In response, those children and young people whose embodiment marks them outside the apparent potential for productive citizenship strive to be inside, strive to be recognised as valuable. What is required of them in the process is that they be ordinary in order to be included. Seeking the security of ordinariness is an understandable response and one that contains some agency as young people attempt to shape their lives and futures. But that situated agency does not take away the additional work they face, made even more difficult if other aspects of their social background further distances them from the valued futures others believe they should aspire to. Therefore, it is important to imagine alternative citizenship possibilities, which are not predicated on matching a set of criteria that will always set particular groups of people apart. The difficulty is that while there have been more calls over the last two decades for children and young people to be given some level of citizenship status, the process of giving such status has got tied up in disputes about capacity, which once again set the terms of inclusion in a way that emphasise disabled children and young people as deficient and other.

Recognising disabled children and young people as citizens

The developments in childhood studies we discussed in Chapter 1 both reflect and have fuelled an interest in the ways in which children can be recipients of rights and citizenship. This work has argued that there is no longer a justification in seeing children as 'citizens in waiting' (Wyness *et al.*, 2004). An important catalyst for the focus on children's rights was the arguments made by childhood studies writers (James *et al.*, 1998) and children's rights campaigners that we should think of children as being a 'minority group' equivalent to women, or people from ethnic minority backgrounds or other marginalised groups. What they are said to share is a history of marginalised status in society due to the oppression and systematic discrimination directed towards them because of their membership of that group. Such an argument switches the focus away from children's development towards the social conditions within which vulnerability is produced (Christensen, 2000). This understanding includes the possibility that social policy initiatives that have sought to protect children, for example from economic exploitation, have also enforced particular understandings of them as in need of protection and in doing so have generated vulnerability (Sealander, 2003; Simpson, 2013) and inhibited, rather than enhanced, opportunities for social participation and recognition.

Initial demands that children's knowledge, expertise and voice should be recognised led to arguments that they should also be the bearers of rights, in particular that they should have access to self-determination. As governments and policy agencies began to respond to calls for children to be recognised as having rights and some form of citizenship, it quickly became incorporated into existing liberal understandings, which emphasise the right of all people to be free, autonomous and independent (Melton, 2008). The most well-known articulation of children as having rights understood in this way is the UN Convention on the Rights of the Child, published in 1989. Amongst various protections the convention argues children should have, it stipulates in Article 12 that:

> State parties shall assure to the child who is capable of forming his or her own views the right to express those views freely in all matters affecting the child, the views of the child being given due weight in accordance with the age and maturity of the child.
>
> (UNICEF, 1989: 5)

What is significant here is how the Convention explicitly connects rights to capacity: 'the child who is capable'. Much of the children's rights legislation that has followed has retained this connection. For example, the UK's Children Act of 1989 includes statements such as:

> Courts should take into account the ascertainable wishes and feelings of the child concerned (considered in the light of his [*sic*] age and understanding).
>
> (Children Act, 1989: Section 1:2)

While the growth of legislation supporting children's rights has been broadly welcomed by children's rights advocates, there are a variety of problems we will discuss here.

The first criticism comes from writers and campaigners working in the Global South who argue that such calls are embedded in Global North depictions of childhood and development. Mechanisms such as the UN Convention are far removed from the realities of the lives of children trying to survive war, absolute poverty and environmental destruction (which are unevenly felt by disabled children and young people in those locations). For example, the Convention is criticised for being unnecessarily grounded in models of child development that reflect Global North values and norms (Boyden, 1997). Freeman (2009: 384) quotes Ncube, a Zimbabwean writer, who notes 'the normative universality achieved in the definition and formulation of children's rights has to contend with diverse and varied cultural and traditional conceptions of childhood, its role, its rights and obligations' (Ncube, 1998: 5). Bühler-Niederberger and Van Krieken (2005: 149) argue that 'contemporary childhoods remain positioned between, on the one hand, modern conceptions of children's rights and, on the other hand, routines and practices that produce and preserve social inequalities'. Woodhead (2009: 51) criticises the World Bank's account of children's development, which for example says that by the age of two children will be able to climb stairs, enjoy stories and wish to claim independence, pointing out that, 'No cultural qualifiers are offered, not even acknowledgement that millions of the world's children may never have seen a staircase, far less had the opportunity to climb one, nor had access to story books. Asserting independence is, moreover, far from universal as a developmental goal'. One example where the tensions between claims to universal rights and recognition of the cultural specificity of the concept of childhood can be seen is in the debates about child labour in the Global South. The child to be saved from economic exploitation is a child created in the imaginary of the Global North who does not speak to or engage with the social and economic practices that place children in the factories, farms, mines and other workplaces of the Global South (Abebe and Bessell, 2011; Hilson, 2012).

What such criticism points to is a concern that the universalist and individualistic imaginaries incorporated into children's rights advocacy will be differentially beneficial, because they do little to challenge inequalities between children and the societies they live in and because they retain a template of childhood, which many children remain outside of. There is a fundamental weakness in such articulations of rights, a weakness of equal significance to disabled children and young people. It leaves unquestioned the rules of the game that set disabled children and young people apart due to their apparent inability to develop correctly and to enact individual citizenship.

The second notable criticism uses the focus on capacity to challenge the wisdom of children's rights. This criticism highlights a difficulty in seeking to use liberal and legalistic approaches that link recognition to the individual capacity to act as a citizen for advocating citizenship for disabled children and young people. It is the apparent inability of disabled children and young people to be capable that has acted as an important barrier to promoting the possibility that they could be thought of as citizens. If individual capacity has to be evident, proposing its absence is an important route through which disabled young people – for their own good – can be said to be outside citizenship. Their apparent vulnerability, due to both their age and their disability, implies that it would be best for others – namely responsible adults – to be the main decision makers in their lives.

Philosophers and political theorists argue that while the notion of rights has an appeal, it risks ignoring the fundamental differences between children and adults (Huntington, 2006). In particular, that developmentally children are at a different stage in life that generates vulnerabilities best protected by others acting on their behalf, rather than passing on to them the responsibilities of citizenship: what Stasiulis (2002) has spoken of as the right to be playful and childish. Cockburn (2013: 137) summarises such arguments as claiming 'children do not have full autonomy, and therefore rights as a mechanism for promotion of their welfare or access to citizenship are ineffective and inappropriate'. This kind of approach seeks to resist the move identified above, which sees children as akin to other 'minority' groups who have been historically and unfairly denied citizenship rights. The argument is that children intrinsically lack capacities that the marginalised groups do have, but which were just denied. Archard usefully summarises the capacity argument:

> Children lack certain cognitive abilities – for example to acquire and to process information in an ordered fashion, to form consistent and stable beliefs, and to appreciate the significance of options and their consequences. They also lack certain volitional abilities – for example, to form, retain and act in the light of consistent desires, and to make independent choices.
>
> (Archard, 2003: 11)

One of the most influential challenges to a focus on rights over protection is the case made by the renowned philosopher O'Neill (1988). In a complex deliberation, she distinguishes between positive rights that are about having access to the protection of law and institutions such as welfare and education, and fundamental rights that are about the right to autonomy and agency due to one's capacity for rationality and moral thought. She argues that children cannot have fundamental rights due to their developmental stage, and that the best way to ensure they acquire positive rights is to ensure that adults, who are capable of exercising fundamental rights, fulfil 'fundamental obligations' towards children on their behalf. Her fear is that a focus on the rights of children does not capture their specific vulnerabilities – 'children's lives are particularly vulnerable to unkindness, to lack of involvement, cheerfulness or good feeling' (O'Neill, 1988: 450). The nature of such vulnerabilities are not protected by rights – 'Cold, distant or fanatical parents and teachers, even if they violate no rights, deny children 'the genial play of life': they can wither children's lives' (O'Neill,

1988: 450–451). Such vulnerabilities come from children's unique dependency, something which is not shared by other 'minority groups'. For these other groups, rights claims are a legitimate response to the oppression they have experienced, as for them arguments that as human beings they should have fundamental rights are an important way to refute previous and ongoing harm. This argument does not work for children because:

> Younger children are completely and unavoidably dependent on those who have power over their lives. Theirs is not a dependence which has been artificially produced (although it can be artificially prolonged); nor can it be ended merely by social or political changes, nor are others reciprocally dependent on children.
>
> (O'Neill, 1988: 461)

While for oppressed groups, accessing rights necessitates challenging those who have produced their oppression and taking away their power, for children their development and growth towards adulthood occurs through those with power over them – parents and carers, and key social institutions such as education – doing their best for children. O'Neill (1988: 463) summarises her argument by suggesting that the best way for children to access the full scope of rights is to 'grow up'. This articulation is a classic formulation of the notion that children are 'not-yet-citizens' (Moosa-Mitha, 2005). The problem is that for disabled children and young people an approach such as this, which focuses on capacity, means that they are in the end thought of as 'never-to-be-citizens' who will not 'grow up' in the way O'Neill imagines.

This focus on vulnerability brings with it dangers. If children are seen as vulnerable simply as children, with an ascending scale that suggests that the older the child, the less vulnerable they are, then we are stuck within an essentialist and developmental approach, which has not learnt from the ideas within childhood studies. It requires the child to – in ways an adult does not have to – prove capacity before consideration is given that they may have a right to be involved in their lives (Ennew, 1994; Freeman, 1997). They remain as 'objects of intervention' (Freeman, 1997: 53) open to exploitation and harm. Whether this be parents or support workers there is good reason to question the assumption that they do know what is best and will simply act in the child's best interests, untouched by their own considerations of what they think is right and their own best interest. As discussed earlier, acting in what they believe to be the child's best interests, parents, carers, and medical actors can pursue painful and invasive treatments geared towards acquiring some proximity to normality. The history of the 'care' of disabled children points to the social production of vulnerability through the denial of any say or freedoms to them in contexts such as residential care. The majority of the asylums of old may have gone, but the legacy of disabled children being treated as essentially vulnerable beings for whom others must act on their behalf, still dominates over more situated appreciations of how they can be brought into decisions about their lives and recognised for having expertise in their own lives. The capacity argument sets up disabled children and young people to fail. It also requires of them that they must at least try to work towards this ideal of how people should be – able, rational, reasoned – trapping them in dynamics of monitoring, disciplining and regulation by institutions of welfare and education seeking to mould them against that template. The risk of associating individual rights with individual capacity is that it justifies the regulatory dynamics we discussed at the beginning of this chapter, which distance children and young people from citizenship rights, rather than enable them.

The way out of the capacity argument is not to assert that all children as individuals do (or could) have enough capacity to be given access to citizenship. This is not to say that disabled children and young people essentially or inevitably lack capacities for agency and participation that others have. Instead, it is to question the value of the individual capacity route as an effective pathway towards recognition and citizenship for children and young people, disabled ones in particular. The problem with capacity is that it requires first a bar to be set and then passed for recognition to be given, without the bar itself being questioned. The inbuilt assumption about what capacities are required and how they are measured are themselves not scrutinised. The way forward is to find better grounds than imaginaries of capacity, understood as the property of an individual self, able to exercise rationality and reason.

The first step in doing so is to seek a way out of the false dichotomy created between children as autonomous independent actors with the same rights as adults, and children as dependent vulnerable subjects under the authority of those who will act in their best interest. Doing so does not ignore that there are a range of differences between adults and children, some of which come from the varied journey from childhood into adulthood. As Freeman (2009: 385) notes:

> To recognise that children's rights are human rights is also to recognise that children are humans, that they are not animals or pieces of property. But this does not mean that we have to overlook the fact that they are also children and, as such, vulnerable.

Instead it is about not seeing vulnerability as leaving one unable to have capacity. As Archard (1993: 61) argues, acknowledging children's particular vulnerabilities as children should not be seen as implying that they have no capacity to challenge and resist such vulnerabilities: 'A child may suffer particular harms because she is a child but may not be, because she is a child, incapable of exercising the rights that protect her against these harms'. It is reasonable to think of childhood as involving particular vulnerabilities that are associated with being young, but within such appreciations we also need to be aware of several factors.

First, as we have seen, many of the vulnerabilities children face are social, including the vulnerabilities that disabled children and young people face in being excluded from society and marginalised due to how others further infantilise them because of their impairments. Second, that some of those experiences make disabled children and young people experts in their lives, able to identify discrimination others are unable (unwilling) to see. Instead, in the words of Garland-Thomson (2011), what the misfit has is epistemic privilege in understanding the world from their perspective. Third, such knowledge and understanding can make them *more* capable, not less, in seeking a say, not just in their own lives, but in the lives of others, calling for change.

From within childhood studies there is a shift towards thinking about capacity in a way that acknowledges both the social construction of childhood and the social relationships that inform children's socio-cultural worlds (Bosisio, 2008; Nieuwenhuys, 2008). Usefully they draw heavily from feminist work on citizenship that advocates for a focus on recognition of difference, relationality and interdependence (Feminist Review, 1997). Such work uses notions of situated agency and interdependence as a way to capture children and young people's relational presence in society and the value there could be in recognising that presence as a basis on which young people can have rights and some say in their lives. Such approaches have much to offer in thinking through disabled children and young people' lives – although interestingly they have not given much consideration to disability (a product we would argue of childhood studies' general lack of consideration of disability).

Relationality and difference

Models of citizenship that see citizens as those able to act autonomously, independently and rationally, are secured in universal values of human rights. Yet their universality does not engage with the fictional nature of such citizenship capacities. They hold autonomy as the key to rights of participation, while not acknowledging its fragility. As Garland-Thomson (1997: 45) argues 'Autonomy assumes immunity to external forces along with the capacity to maintain a stable, static state of being'. Feminist work on citizenship, which rejects liberal accounts of rights, has been crucial in developing ways to strip away the universality of such citizenship tropes and in producing alternative ways in which to draw difference and relationality into accounts of who can be citizens and what kind of citizenship can be made possible (Brown, 1993). This is clearly a useful resource for us in thinking through how relationality, rather than individual autonomy, can be drawn into a re-categorisation of what makes citizenship possible, particularly for disabled children and young people. Recognition of differences is favoured over abstract universalism as the only way in which inequalities in opportunities to enact citizenship can be disturbed and redistributed (Fraser, 1997). Phillips (1993) argues that rights arguments which focus on the abstract individual guarantee that the conditions that generate inequalities are ignored in the apparent pursuit of rights for everyone. Feminists have proposed instead a re-orientation towards thinking of citizens as embedded in practices of community that inform who they are, and which – potentially – are the source of their capacity to act and be recognised (Yuval-Davis, 1997, 2011). Individuals are de-centred by recognising the ways in which lives are 'inescapably part of particular communities and contexts, and the values embedded there help us to set goals for ourselves' (Rudy, 1999: 48). Our embeddedness in community means that there 'is no pre-social component because the self is always situated within a concrete set of circumstances, beliefs, and constructions' (Rudy, 1999: 48).

This work is now being used to advocate for children as citizens and to challenge the accounts above which see protection, vulnerability and reduced capacity as justifications for viewing citizenship as a concept not helpful for children. This is where the benefit of seeing citizenship as a range of practices broader than that which occurs between state and the individual becomes visible. We are not just citizens when we are formally recognised by the state. We are also citizens when we participate in the social world and in particular when that participation makes a difference to our life and the lives of others. Various writers have argued that formal understandings of citizenship acts will always disadvantage children as they are unable to fulfil such duties (Jans, 2004; Larkins, 2014). Instead, this work is much more focused on social rights and citizenship. Crucially, it is also centred on analysing and recognising the relationships children are in as vital components in either enabling them – with others – to enact citizenship or being blocked from such possibilities:

> Rather than passive recipients of the legal status of citizenship, conveyed by nation-states, in difference-centred approaches, citizens define citizenship through practices and in relationship with others and communities.
>
> (Larkins, 2014: 9)

Larkins argues it is more productive to focus on the horizontal dimensions of social engagement and the possibilities of citizenship activity there, than to always consider the relationship between state and individual, which inevitably fall into discussions of rights and responsibilities and the abstraction of law. Through the relationships that form in social interaction, people – including children and those around them – can (while not always) live out transgressive ways in which to be a citizen.

The work of Lister (1997) provides an important and useful bridge between these feminist approaches and the advocacy of rights for children and young people. For Lister, what makes something an act of citizenship is not where it takes place – public or private – but the public consequences of the act. This can therefore include the private acts of care that women provide, which fall into the public sphere through the demand they can make for welfare and the state to act differently. Such care acts also project a different form of human activity focused on interdependency and care, rather than individual accomplishment and perseverance (Lister, 2007a). Lister's work on women and citizenship has consistently argued that uniform definitions and measures of citizenship will always be exclusionary for some by failing to recognise the structurally different lives people live because of their gender. The only way to enable full citizenship for women is to both recognise the ways in which they are citizens that differ from men – via their political acts associated with their involvement in care – and in the specific challenges they face in accessing rights to citizenship – via the assumptions made that they are less rational than men, weaker and more prone to act with emotion rather than reason. Lister has drawn this difference argument into an account of children by proposing: 'that the criteria for inclusion as citizens cannot be uniform and, for the same reason that they cannot be modelled on male norms, so they [citizenship rights for children] cannot be modelled on adult norms' (Lister, 2007b: 716). Her approach does not require that children be citizens in all aspects that are the same as adults; this is an unfair and unreasonable obligation that is not necessary in order to say that they can and should have opportunities to be involved in citizenship practice. This form of 'lived citizenship', she argues, is a better starting point for advocating for citizenship rights for children. If the focus is on enabling children to participate in their communities and institutions, then it should not be contingent on them proving – to the judgement of others – that they can participate in the same way and to the same level as adults. Dichotomous thinking that places immaturity in opposition to maturity is too open to discriminatory judgements, as has been and still is directed towards women, to act as a measure of the rights to citizenship.

Moosa-Mitha (2005) has drawn heavily upon the ideas of Lister to develop an approach to children and young people's citizenship that incorporates difference as a framing concept. In the way that Lister argues for gender differences being acknowledged in order for women to acquire genuine citizenship, Moosa-Mitha argues that what makes children different from adults should be the key to their citizenship, rather than the rationale for denying it to them. She sees childhood as a distinct stage of life, but not one defined by lack and a need to prepare for future citizenship:

> Difference-centred models would posit the child as having an 'active' self – one that has agency. Thus children may not be responsible for how the world is, and they may not have the psychological wherewithal to make 'rational choices' but they certainly respond, mitigate, resist, have views about and interact with the social conditions in which they find themselves.
>
> (Moosa-Mitha, 2005: 380)

Like Larkin, she moves away from a focus on the agency exercised between the individual and the state towards recognition of the everyday relational agency children are capable of having within their lives. Her focus is on children and young people as having a 'presence' in their communities, and it is this presence and the difference they make through it, which should be acknowledged and legitimated:

> I would re-define children's rights of freedom, in this associational sense, by examining if children are able to have a presence in the many relationships in which they participate. By presence, I mean the degree to which the voice, contribution and agency of the child is acknowledged in their many

relationships. Presence, more than autonomy, acknowledges the self as relational and dialogical, thereby suggesting that it is not enough to have a voice, it is equally important to also be heard in order for one to have a presence in society.

(Moosa-Mitha, 2005: 381)

This concentration on recognising what children are already part of and doing generates a more emancipatory and generous imaginary seeking to find ways to increase children's presence and to advocate for relational opportunities within which they can thrive. It is within relationships that children's agency can develop and grow. Such agency does not need to reach the high standards asked by those who question children's capacity for citizenship status, while also recognising the relational and contingent nature of all people's ability and wish to participate in things that matter to them. Participation is re-imagined as something that people engage each other with, rather than a tactic of the individual to ensure they excel against others.

Relational and situated understandings of capacity have been used by a variety of researchers examining the potential for children to have presence in their lives and the lives of others, even in contexts of oppression and significant hardship, including in the Global South. A range of writers and activists have called for greater recognition of the capacity of children living in extraordinarily difficult situations to be active agents (often at great risk) in challenging their situation and changing their lives and the lives of those around them. For example, in research on children workers and campaigners, Liebel (2003) argues that through working together on campaigns to improve their working conditions (rather than be removed from the workplace) they are 'subjects of rights' in their nations. Their capacities to generate change are:

> primarily founded on their own experience, and are immediately related to the realities of their lives. They are not formulae of compromise or general principles that leave broad, almost unlimited scope for interpretation, but concrete programmes of action in experienced or conceivable situations in life.
>
> (quoted in Cockburn 2013: 199–200 (Liebel, 2003: 188))

Thinking of disabled children and young people as 'subjects of rights', present in the social world, with an interest and a right to have a say in it, is clearly something worth exploring.

Disabled children and young people as subjects of rights

Relational and difference-centred approaches to citizenship have the potential to offer more expansive terms to both recognise the capacities of disabled children and young people, and to push for the opportunities for them to enact those capacities. They also appear to offer ways to counter dynamics of monitoring, regulation and social control, which are justified by seeking to normalise the capacities of disabled children and young people in order for them to be recognised as possible future citizens. However, some important issues need to be resolved first.

Across the book we have argued that disabled children and young people are relational actors embedded in the multiple networks they help shape and which inform their identities and practices. However, in recognising the importance of these relationships we have acknowledged that the relationships disabled children and young people are in with peers, friends, family, social others, and formal providers of support are not always positive and can be the source of regulatory monitoring. We have discussed that we should not assume that the adults around disabled children and young people know and assert their best interests: instead they can be key actors trying to normalise and control their presence. We have seen how those closest to them can advocate for the surgeries and changes to behaviour required of them in order to mimic the normality that conditions their social recognition. Therefore, not all relationships and actions made possible by others produce a counterbalance to normality and a willingness to embrace difference. Finally, we have also highlighted across the book that much of the work of trying to appear effortlessly normal and ordinary is done as the price of membership of broader communities; whether that be the classroom, the friendship group, the pub or broader spaces of the public realm. Such work implies communities where belonging is conditional and prescriptive rather than embracing and welcoming.

Therefore, in proposing that disabled children and young people can be citizens via the social and personal relationships and communities they are part of, we need to add it is those relationships and communities that embrace their differences and their misfit qualities which will enable this. This is possible because communities, as well as being barriers to recognition due to their rules of inclusion, can be challenged, remade. Holt *et al.* (2013) argue that the micro dynamics of contemporary segregation do have within them the space necessary for challenge and resistance. Yuvul-Davis (1997: 8) suggests such challenge often comes via the actions of those a community tries to deny entry: 'Collectivities and 'communities' are ideological and material constructions, whose boundaries, structures and norms are a result of constant processes of struggles'. Through their engagement with communities and their efforts to remake them – efforts we can think of as acts of citizenship – disabled children and young people can be participants in the 'struggles around the determination of what is involved in belonging, in being a member of a community' (Yuval-Davis, 2011: 27). These acts of citizenship occur within disabled children and young people's active presence in social interactions where embodied differences are visible, welcomed and acknowledged as valued ways to be human.

Across our projects we have seen relational acts of resistance that challenge the boundaries of community recognition and make expansive spaces for embodied difference within those communities. Family and friends, teachers and medical actors are partners in resistance and advocates of social citizenship when they push others to recognise difference as a contribution to social life, rather than merely inconvenient or uncomfortable. When disabled children and young people and others refuse to hide the cooperative and relational labour that is involved in participating in their social worlds they negate normative templates and open up imaginaries for different modes of interaction, space and relationship. Everyday examples include practices such as everyone in a nursery learning Makaton so that communication is done in non-dominating and expansive ways. Or when a child's assistive device becomes a valued part of their identity and offers new and recognised ways to be a social participant. It is when a child's own experiences of pain and the limitations their impairments generate becomes the basis of providing support to others facing difficulty. We have seen parents, significant others, including formal care providers, and disabled children and young people involved in such activities seeking to articulate different versions of community belonging, which are templates of diversity rather than normality. Refusals to explain and justify difference, to challenge the laughter of others, provide cracks in current formulations of human recognition and are part of the agency and citizenship of disabled children and young people. In the *Enabling Care* project we saw parents, including those living in some of the most socially difficult circumstances, participate in activities with others to challenge the communities around them to recognise their children as valued members. In the *Genetic Journeys* project we saw parents refuse to have their lives and the lives of their children disvalued by others. Finally, in the *Embodied Transitions* project we saw young people seek both to belong and to challenge the basis on which they could belong.

At the centre of many of the relational practices we have highlighted, which offer everyday versions of social citizenship involving disabled children and young people and others, is a particular approach to, and understanding of, care. Care has been a troubling concept in disability studies, understandably so given the associations with charity and passivity (Shakespeare, 2006). But the modes of care we are documenting here are not within that framework and are instead deeply political, relational and rooted in values of recognition, partnership and interdependency. For us, they offer a counterbalance to the notion of vulnerability as something both specific to disabled children and young people and a justification for the narrowing of opportunities for citizenship. Instead, the care practices disabled children and young people participate in, which emerge from both their embodied differences and the difficulties of interacting in unwelcoming and unresponsive social and cultural spaces, is central to their citizenship possibilities. What we have in mind are examples such as informal carers resisting the conditions placed on them and their child's recognition by state welfare. Such acts are a challenge to the contemporary withdrawal of formal care; a challenge that is made because of the dis-valuing of the child's different life such withdrawal implies. These practices of care re-position dependency as within, rather than outside of, citizenship practice (Levine, 2005; Lister, 1997; Sevenhuijsen, 1998). It re-orients care as something that emerges from the 'reciprocal dependencies' (Fine and Glendinning, 2005: 616) or 'mutual vulnerability'

(Baier, 1995) inherent in the human condition and denied by false models of individuality and autonomy. Depending on others becomes a part of capacity, rather than evidence of its absence. The participation of disabled children and young people in society, enabled by their relational actions with others, is testament to such 'mutual vulnerability'. Their acts of citizenship therefore emerge from their embodied differences and the interactions that emerge through and with others. Gibson (2006) uses a concept of 'connectivities' to signify what others might think of as the dependencies disabled young people have on others, but which could instead be thought of as positive aspects of their presence and potential in the world. If this understanding is taken into thinking about citizenship, the focus becomes less about achieving a mythical autonomy and independence no one can achieve and instead more about recognising such connectivities as valued forms of being that reflect the interdependencies we all share, and creating institutional and social contexts that can enable them to flourish (Gibson *et al.*, 2012).

Conclusion

Citizenship ideas always, reasonably, include discussion of responsibility; that to have the rights of citizenship, the holder also carries certain responsibilities. The conditionality of contemporary citizenship could be thought of in the same way, to have these rights citizens should abide by these conditions. The problem is that the conditions we see articulated in neo-liberal states are problematically limiting the possibilities for a variety of groups to gain entry and remain within citizenship. The only way disabled people can comply with such conditions is to overcome their disabilities. This is what we have seen many disabled children and young people strive to do, in order to be granted entry into the social world, now and in the future. This leaves their citizenship contingent on the compliance of their minds-bodies with such requirements and is a source of far more vulnerability than their own minds-bodies produce.

The inequalities and vulnerabilities produced by contemporary conditionality require a response and disabled children and young people, like other marginalised groups, are involved in producing that response. It is a response that emerges in social practice, it requires different imaginaries too, which emerge from the coming together of narrative with interaction. The social practices we have witnessed provide clues to the different types of communities, institutions and cultural understandings, which could provide the spaces within which differences of a variety of types could have a presence not reliant on minimal hospitality and the allowances of others.

It begins with not assuming disabled children and young people are either essentially vulnerable or capable, but become so through the actions and inactions of others. The promise of capacity lies in the relational properties of the worlds within which disabled children and young people live. This calls, then, for different ways in which those worlds operate so that differences can be engaged with through better imaginaries. This is not about saying that embodied differences are irrelevant, they are relevant, but not in a way that is about making allowances for them. Instead, it is about the relational agency possible through incorporating them into the social as an intrinsic part of the human condition: perhaps the one thing we all share – bodies of varied and always changing relational capacity.

References

Abebe, T. and Bessell, S. (2011) Dominant discourses, debates and silences on child labour in Africa and Asia. *Third World Quarterly*, 32(4): 765–786.

Archard, D. (1993) *Children: Rights and Childhood*. London: Routledge.

Archard, D. (2003) *Children, Family and the State*. Aldershot: Ashgate.

Bacchi, C.L. and Beasley, C. (2002) Citizen bodies: is embodied citizenship a contradiction in terms? *Critical Social Policy*, 22(2): 324–352.

Baier, A.C. (1995) *Moral Prejudice*. London: Harvard University Press.

Bosisio, R. (2008) 'Right' and 'not right': representations of justice in young people. *Childhood*, 15(2): 276–294.

Boyden, J. (1997) Childhood and the policy-makers: a comparative perspective on the globalization of childhood. In A. James and A. Prout (eds), *Constructing and Reconstructing Childhood*. pp. 190–229. London: Falmer Press.

Brown, W. (1993) Wounded attachments. *Political Theory*, 21(3): 390–410.

Bühler-Niederberger, D. and Van Krieken, R. (2005) Persisting inequalities: childhood between global influences and local traditions. *Childhood*, 15(2): 147–155.

Charmaz, K. (1995) The body, identity, and self: adapting to impairment. *Sociological Quarterly*, 36(4): 657–680.

Charmaz, K. (2002) Stories and silences: disclosures and self in chronic illness. *Qualitative Inquiry*, 8(3): 302–328.

Children Act. (1989) *Children Act*. www.legislation.gov.uk/ukpga/1989/41/section/1

Christensen, P. (2000) Childhood and the cultural constitution of vulnerable bodies. In A. Prout (ed.), *The Body, Childhood and Society*. pp. 38–59. Basingstoke: Palgrave.

Cockburn, T. (2013) *Rethinking Children's Citizenship*. Basingstoke: Palgrave Macmillan.

Cohen, E.F. and Morley, C.P. (2009) Children, ADHD, and citizenship. *Journal of Medicine and Philosophy*, 34(2): 155–180.

Dietz, M.G. (1987) Context is all: feminism and theories of citizenship. *Daedalus*, 116(4): 1–24.

Dwyer, P. (2004a) Creeping conditionality in the UK: from welfare rights to conditional entitlements? *Canadian Journal of Sociology*, 29(2): 265–287.

Dwyer, P. (2004b) *Understanding Social Citizenship: Themes and Perspectives for Social Policy*. Bristol: Policy Press.

Ennew, J. (1994) Time for children or for adults. In J. Qvortrup, M. Bardy, G. Sgritta and H. Wintersberger (eds), *Childhood Matters: Social Theory, Practice and Politics*. pp. 125–143. Aldershot: Ashgate.

Enright, M. (2011) Girl interrupted: citizenship and the Irish hijab debate. *Social & Legal Studies*, 20(4): 463–480.

Feminist Review (1997) Citizenship: pushing the boundaries. *Feminist Review*, 57(Autumn).

Fine, M. and Glendinning, C. (2005) Dependence, independence or inter-dependence? Revisiting the concepts of 'care' and 'dependency'. *Ageing & Society*, 25: 601–621.

Fitzpatrick, T. (2001) Before the cradle: new genetics, biopolicy and regulated eugenics. *Journal of Social Policy*, 30: 589–612.

Fraser, N. (1997) *Justice Interruptus: Critical Reflections on the 'Postsocialist' Condition*. London: Routledge.

Fraser, N. and Gordon, L. (1994) Civil citizenship against social citizenship? On the ideology of contract-versus-charity. In B. Van Steenbergen (ed.), *The Condition of Citizenship*. pp. 90–107. London: Sage.

Freeman, M. (1997) *The Moral Status of Children*. Dordrecht, Netherlands: Martinus Nijhoff Publishers.

Freeman, M. (2009) Children's rights as human rights: reading the UNCRC. In J. Qvortrup, W.A. Corsaro and M.-S. Honig (eds), *The Palgrave Handbook of Childhood Studies*. pp. 377–393. Basingstoke: Palgrave Macmillan.

Galvin, R. (2003) The paradox of disability culture: the need to combine versus the imperative to let go. *Disability & Society*, 18(5): 675–690.

Garland-Thomson, R. (1997) *Extraordinary Bodies: Figuring Physical Disability in American Culture and Literature*. New York, NY: New York University Press.

Garland-Thomson, R. (2011) Misfits: a feminist materialist disability concept. *Hypatia – a Journal of Feminist Philosophy*, 26(3): 591–609.

Garland, D. (2001) *The Culture of Control: Crime and Social Order in Contemporary Society*. Oxford: Oxford University Press.

Gibson, B.E. (2006) Disability, connectivity and transgressing the autonomous body. *Journal of Medical Humanities*, 27: 187–196.

Gibson, B.E., Carnevale, F.A. and King, G. (2012) 'This is my way': reimagining disability, in/dependence and interconnectedness of persons and assistive technologies. *Disability and Rehabilitation*, 34(22): 1894–1899.

Hilson, G. (2012) Family hardship and cultural values: child labor in Malian small-scale gold mining communities. *World Development*, 40(8): 1663–1674.

Hindess, B. (2002) Neo-liberal citizenship. *Citizenship Studies*, 6(2): 127–143.

Holt, L., Bowlby, S. and Lea, J. (2013) Emotions and the habitus: young people with socio-emotional differences (re)producing social, emotional and cultural capital in family and leisure space-times. *Emotion, Space and Society*, 9(Nov.): 33–41.

Holt, L., Lea, J. and Bowlby, S. (2012) Special units for young people on the autistic spectrum in mainstream schools: sites of normalisation, abnormalisation, inclusion, and exclusion. *Environment and Planning A*, 44: 2191–2206.

Huntington, C. (2006) Rights myopia in child welfare. *UCLA Law Review*, 53: 637–699.

James, A., Jenks, C. and Prout, A. (1998) *Theorizing Childhood*. Cambridge: Polity Press.

Jamieson, J. (2012) Bleak times for children? The anti-social behaviour agenda and the criminalization of social policy. *Social Policy & Administration*, 46(4): 448–464.

Jans, M. (2004) Children as citizens: towards a contemporary notion of child participation. *Childhood*, 11(1): 27–44.

Kofman, E. (1995) Citizenship for some but not for others: spaces of citizenship in contemporary Europe. *Political Geography*, 14(2): 121–137.

Larkins, C. (2014) Enacting children's citizenship: developing understandings of how children enact themselves as citizens through actions and acts of citizenship *Childhood*, 21(1): 7–21.

Levine, C. (2005) Acceptance, avoidance, and ambiguity: conflicting social values about childhood disability. *Kennedy Institute of Ethics Journal*, 15(4): 371–383.

Lewis, J. (1980) *The Politics of Motherhood*. London: Croom Helm.

Liebel, M. (2003) Working children as social subjects: the contribution of working children's organizations to social transformations. *Childhood*, 10(3): 265–286.

Lister, R. (1997) *Citizenship: Feminist Perspectives*. Basingstoke: Macmillan.

Lister, R. (2007a) Inclusive citizenship: realizing potential. *Citizenship Studies*, 11(1): 49–61.

Lister, R. (2007b) Why citizenship? Where, when and how children? *Theoretical Inquiries in Law*, 8: 693–718.

MacDonald, R. (1997) *Youth, the 'Underclass' and Social Exclusion*. London: Routledge.

Marshall, T.H. (1950) *Citizenship and Social Class: And Other Essays*. Cambridge: Cambridge University Press.

McLaughlin, J., Phillimore, P. and Richardson, D. (eds) (2011) *Contesting Recognition: Culture, Identity and Citizenship*. Basingstoke: Palgrave Macmillan.

Melton, G.B. (2008) Beyond balancing: toward an integrated approach to children's rights. *Journal of Social Issues*, 64(4): 903–920.

Moosa-Mitha, M. (2005) A difference-centred alternative to theorization of children's citizenship rights. *Citizenship Studies*, 9(4): 369–388.

Muncie, J. (2006) Governing young people: coherence and contradiction in contemporary youth justice. *Critical Social Policy*, 26(4): 770–793.

Ncube, W. (1998) Prospects and challenges in Eastern and Southern Africa: the interplay between international human rights norms and domestic law, tradition and law. In W. Ncube (ed.), *Law, Culture, Tradition and Children's Rights in Eastern and Southern Africa*. pp. 1–10. Dartmouth: Ashgate.

Nieuwenhuys, O. (2008) Editorial: the ethics of children's rights. *Childhood*, 15(1): 4–11.

O'Neill, O. (1988) Children's rights and children's lives. *Ethics, Place and Environment*, 98(3): 445–463.

Oliver, M. (1996) *Understanding Disability: From Theory to Practice*. London: Macmillan.

Ouellette, A. (2010) Shaping parental authority over children's bodies. *Indiana Law Journal*, 85(3): 955–1002.

Phillips, A. (1993) *Democracy and Difference*. Cambridge: Polity Press.

Rudy, K. (1999) Liberal theory and feminist politics. *Women and Politics*, 20(2): 33–57.

Scully, J.L. (2010) Hidden labor: disabled/nondisabled encounters, agency and autonomy. *International Journal of Feminist Approaches to Bioethics*, 3(2): 25–42.

Sealander, J. (2003) *The Failed Century of the Child*. Cambridge: Cambridge University Press.

Sevenhuijsen, S. (1998) *Citizenship and the Ethics of Care*. London: Routledge.

Shakespeare, T. (2006) *Disability Rights and Wrongs*. London: Routledge.

Shildrick, M. (2005) Transgressing the law with Foucault and Derrida: some reflections on anomalous embodiment. *Critical Quarterly*, 47(3): 30–46.

Silvers, A. and Francis, L.P. (2005) Justice through trust: disability and the 'outlier problem' in social contract theory. *Ethics*, 116(1): 40–76.

Simpson, B. (2013) Challenging childhood, challenging children: children's rights and sexting. *Sexualities*, 16(5–6): 690–709.

Stasiulis, D. (2002) The active child citizen: lessons from Canadian policy and children's movement. *Citizenship Studies*, 6(4): 507–538.

Turner, B.S. (ed.) (2000a) *Citizenship and Social Theory*. London: Sage.

Turner, B.S. (2000b) Contemporary problems in the theory of citizenship. In B.S. Turner (ed.), *Citizenship and Social Theory*. pp. 1–18. London: Sage.

UNICEF (1989) *UN Convention on the Rights of the Child*. New York, NY: UNICEF.

van Steenbergen, B. (1994) The condition of citizenship: an introduction. In B. van Steen-bergen (ed.), *The Condition of Citizenship*. pp. 1–9. London: Sage.

Williams, F. (2008) Culture and nationhood. In P. Alcock, A. Erskine, M. May and K. Rowlingson (eds), *The Student's Companion to Social Policy*. pp. 146–152. London: Blackwell.

Woodhead, M. (2009) Child development and the development of childhood. In J. Qvor-trup, W.A. Corsaro and M.-S. Honig (eds), *The Palgrave Handbook of Childhood Studies*. pp. 46–61. Basingstoke: Palgrave Macmillan.

Wyness, M., Harrison, L. and Buchanan, I. (2004) Childhood, politics and ambiguity: towards an agenda for children's political inclusion. *Sociology*, 38(1): 81–99.

Yuval-Davis, N. (1991) The citizenship debate: women, ethnic processes and the State. *Feminist Review*, 39(Autumn): 58–68.

Yuval-Davis, N. (1997) Women, citizenship and difference. *Feminist Review*, 57: 4–27.

Yuval-Davis, N. (2011) Belonging and the politics of belonging. In J. McLaughlin, P. Phillimore and D. Richardson (eds), *Contesting Recognition: Culture, Identity and Citizenship*. pp. 20–35. Basingstoke: Palgrave.

Index

For Product Safety Concerns and Information please contact our EU
representative GPSR@taylorandfrancis.com
Taylor & Francis Verlag GmbH, Kaufingerstraße 24, 80331 München, Germany

www.ingramcontent.com/pod-product-compliance
Ingram Content Group UK Ltd.
Pitfield, Milton Keynes, MK11 3LW, UK
UKHW020952180425
457613UK00019B/634